Never Put a Cactus in the Bathroom

Never
Put a Cactus in the
Bathroom

A ROOM-BY-ROOM GUIDE TO
STYLING AND CARING FOR
YOUR HOUSEPLANTS

Emily L. Hay Hinsdale
Illustrations by Loni Harris

TILLER PRESS

NEW YORK   LONDON   TORONTO   SYDNEY   NEW DELHI

TILLER PRESS

An Imprint of Simon & Schuster, Inc.
1230 Avenue of the Americas
New York, NY 10020

Copyright © 2021 by Simon & Schuster, Inc.

All rights reserved, including the right to reproduce this book or portions
thereof in any form whatsoever. For information, address Simon & Schuster
Subsidiary Rights Department, 1230 Avenue of the Americas, New York, NY 10020.

First Tiller Press hardcover edition April 2021

TILLER PRESS and colophon are trademarks of Simon & Schuster, Inc.

For information about special discounts for bulk purchases, please
contact Simon & Schuster Special Sales at 1-866-506-1949
or business@simonandschuster.com.

The Simon & Schuster Speakers Bureau can bring authors to your live event.
For more information or to book an event, contact the Simon & Schuster Speakers
Bureau at 1-866-248-3049 or visit our website at www.simonspeakers.com.

Interior design by Laura Levatino
Illustrations by Loni Harris

Manufactured in China

3   5   7   9   10   8   6   4

Library of Congress Cataloging-in-Publication Data has been applied for.

ISBN 978-1-9821-6583-3
ISBN 978-1-9821-6584-0 (ebook)

For Bill, Clara, and Rose, who help me grow

Contents

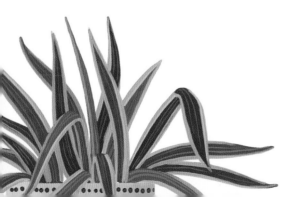

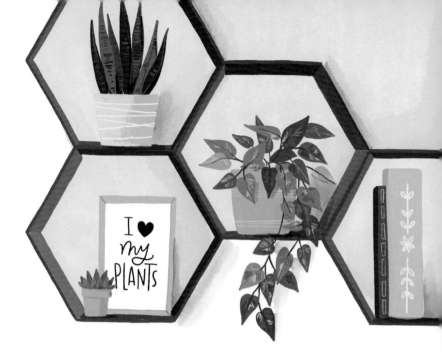

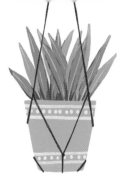

Never Put a Cactus in the Bathroom

Part 1

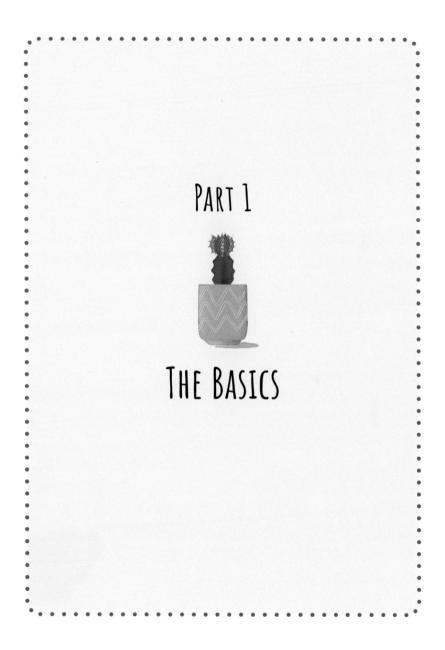

The Basics

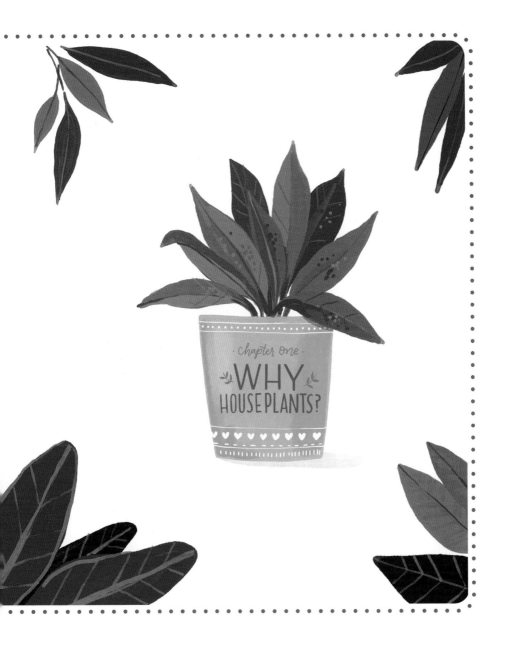

chapter one

WHY
HOUSE PLANTS?

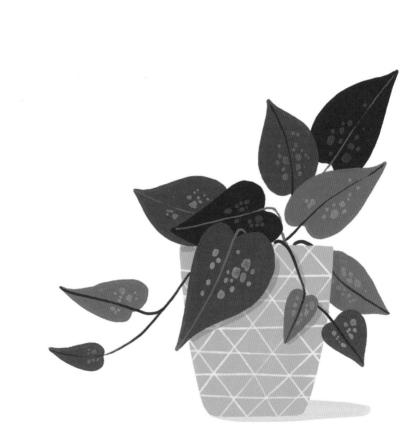

ou remember your first houseplant—the terrarium you made in fourth grade, the pot of ivy on your college dorm windowsill, the philodendron your grandma gave you for your first apartment, the orchid that lasted longer than the ex who bought it for you. At first, you cherished that special plant and watered it meticulously and gave it a place of pride in your space. But you know you weren't committed. You weren't ready. The terrarium started to smell, the ivy got lost when you moved dorms, the philodendron turned yellow, and you threw out that orchid when it lost its bloom.

But now you are ready for the real thing: plant parenthood. You understand that like that ivy, you have outgrown the confines of a small and humdrum space and are ready to introduce some physically and mentally refreshing green energy into your home, your office, and your life. Whether this is your first sprout or your passion for houseplants is in full bloom, it's time to dig into some dirt about growing your space into a happy green home.

Fortunately, your timing is good. This is not the era (cough, 1970s) of the ubiquitous grocery store African violet sitting under fluorescent lights. These days our plants can feature prominently in our plans to do better by ourselves: while you find the light in your life, so, too, can you work to find the right light to help your little vine twine.

Houseplant popularity ebbs and flows with fashion through history, but at each budding of indoor-plant enthusiasm, plants seem to take on a symbolic meaning. For example, three thousand years ago, the Chinese started growing ornamental plants indoors as a sign of wealth. Tending a miniature flowering azalea during the winter certainly suggests a life of leisure! The legendary Hanging Gardens of Babylon were supposedly an extravagant gift of love from a king to a queen who missed her greener homeland. When Christopher Columbus (and other early Western explorers) sailed the ocean blue in 1492, he brought home tropical plants from new lands, a living history of exploration. The Victorians favored hearty plants like aspidistras that could survive the drafty, dim houses and polluted atmosphere—unsurprising in an era that had only just discovered central heating—more elaborate houseplants were a sign that amateur botanists' quality of life was on the way up. The mid-twentieth century introduced the idea of plants as room-by-room decor, and spider plants draped over living room TV cabinets, while philodendrons popped up in office cubicles.

Recent trends move raising houseplants beyond the purely decorative to discovering how even a little indoor greenery supports our physical and mental wellness. This is a time period when we're learning that nurturing our individual well-being translates into contributing more positively to our whole society—working better, living better, being better. We're turning over a new leaf.

Now that you know a plant for your home is a great way to go, how do you find the right one?

Why Houseplants?

Any home-decorating magazine will feature spreads of fabulous fiddle-leaf fig trees and dazzling dracaenas. While these plants did a great job being trucked in for a day's photo shoot, when you're planning a longer-term houseplant relationship, you'll need to spend some time making sure it's the right plant for you. Are you a novice already feeling a little nervous after all these mentions of philodendrons and violets? Start with something low-maintenance and reliable. Did you keep that ivy from college alive after all? You may be ready to tackle a more touchy plant like a bromeliad. Do you love the exotic and dramatic? A hanging display of air plants might make an interesting addition to your space. Are you more practical in your home-decorating interests? A selection of kitchen herbs can be an attractive and delicious way to save money on grocery store herb bunches.

There are perfect plants for every level of indoor gardener and every room in your home.

In the pages that follow, we'll talk about understanding the quality of daylight in your home. We'll review how to get started in identifying the way to properly pot and display any plant. You'll learn about danger signs to watch for in a sick plant, like drooping or yellow leaves, and how to know which plants will work with the other members of your household, human or animal. We'll make some recommendations for how to fit your plant into your decor and the use of different spaces—sun-loving plants for warm windowsills, water-loving plants for humid areas, and even plants that thrive in a dim, neglected corner.

Once you know what you can do for your plant, take a look at what your plant can do for you.

Healthier Air

It's not an exaggeration or a flower child's dream to say that houseplants improve air quality. You may or may not remember your high school science class explanations of plant respiration. Here's the short version: while humans breathe in oxygen and breathe out carbon dioxide, plants absorb carbon dioxide and produce oxygen. The perfect pair.

Having a few of these little oxygen factories in your home will constantly replenish your personal atmosphere, pumping clean, refreshed air to your brain and body to support your overall health. (But don't worry, if you can't make things work with your fern, you'll still be able to breathe!)

Beyond the symbiosis of plant and animal life, plants are natural filters for many toxins that pervade our environment, especially enclosed indoor spaces. In a 1989 study, NASA demonstrated that certain kinds of plants can filter the following common "sick building" by-products of cleaning materials, printing ink, paint, and other toxins from our air:

- trichloroethylene (can cause dizziness, headaches, nausea, and vomiting)
- formaldehyde (can cause irritation to the nose, mouth, and throat, and in severe cases, swelling of the larynx and lungs)
- benzene (can cause irritation to the eyes, dizziness, headaches, confusion, and drowsiness)

- xylene (can cause irritation to the mouth and throat, heart problems, headaches, and dizziness)
- ammonia (can cause eye irritation, coughing, and sore throat)

While NASA's study focused on small indoor spaces (like a spaceship?) and shouldn't be taken as proof that plants eliminate *all* unhealthy atmospheres, the prospect of not breathing toxins seems like a good reason to cuddle up to a chrysanthemum.

> NASA recommended at least one plant for every hundred square feet. You wouldn't want to argue with NASA, would you?

HEATHIER MIND

Why do studies show that people perform better when they're working and living around plants? Maybe because we grew up together—animal world and plant world—and your childhood friends can put you at ease. Or maybe it's because your cactus is better looking than your coworkers.

Whatever the reason, several studies have demonstrated higher and better productivity when people share their space with plants. Offices with plant decor see as much as 40 percent higher worker happiness and productivity (I'm not sure how to measure happiness, but apparently it's about the size of a jade plant). Schools that added plants to classrooms saw a rise in children's test scores. Hospital patients with green plants instead of just sickly green wall paint have a faster recovery time.

If you need a brain boost to get through the day, just buddy up with a begonia.

Healthier Spirit

Close your eyes and go to your happy place. It's probably a different spot for each of us, but psychologists report that for most of us, it's somewhere in nature—a beach, a lake, a forest, a garden. So why is it that we spend the majority of our day looking at a view that mostly includes walls and furniture (on average, people spend 90 percent of their day inside)? Bringing a little nature indoors is like bringing meditation into your every moment.

Beyond just the positive benefits of being around plants, the act of maintaining houseplants can be a thoughtful experience. Watering, dusting, and pruning your indoor plant friends isn't something you can hurry through in order to check it off your list. It requires patience and diligence. Tend to your plants with peace and focus, and plant care can become a meditation in and of itself.

When you're stressed or overwhelmed, take a deep breath, exhale, and listen to your snake plant breathe it in.

Know Your Houseplant

Let's start with some quick definitions for the houseplant newbie.

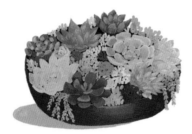

Succulents

You've probably seen a million of these, since they are some of the most popular indoor plants. They can be small enough to fit in your palm, and their neat edges and patterns give them an appealing decorative, sculptural appearance. They are so perfect-looking that they're the models for some of the more successful fake plant varieties available by the dozen at Ikea. But nothing beats the real thing.

Succulents get their name from juicy, fleshy stems and leaves, their way of retaining water in drier climates or when you forget to water them. These are great starter plants because they take some effort to kill. Look for jade plants, hens and chicks, aloe vera, and zebra plants to start.

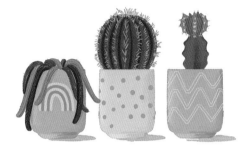

Cacti

Most cacti are a kind of succulent, similarly built to retain water in dry environments. But unlike previously mentioned succulents, cacti have largely given up the leafy look, opting instead for a predator-discouraging, water-loss-reducing, spiny aspect. There is a huge variety of cacti, from the forty-foot saguaro to the fruit-producing prickly pear. Moving indoors to a perhaps more sensible size, there are still dozens of cacti at your disposal, like the barrel cactus, moon cactus, or flowering Christmas cactus. Actually, saguaros and prickly pears in a more compact form both work indoors, too. It won't be a surprise that these desert natives like lots of sun, warm windows, and only occasional watering.

Just be thoughtful where you place these houseplants. A cactus is a terrible acquaintance to run into in a dark room in the middle of the night.

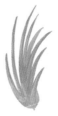

Air Plants

These are the odd little clusters of what looks spiky hair. In fact, sometimes they're sold atop small statues for a gray-green punk rock look. Very weird. Air plants (*Tillandsia*) are a kind of epiphyte, which means they like to attach to other plants rather than root in soil. They like indirect light, so find a place for them with a window nearby, but not one that floods with enough sunshine to heat the room. These are tropical plants and they absorb a lot of the water they need straight from the air. Bathrooms, where the shower steam that may fog your mirror will keep your air plant extra happy, make a great home for them. In less humid locations, infrequent watering is necessary. Give it a good soak, dry it out, and release it back into the air.

Air plants are really fun to display in inventive ways, since they don't require bulky pots. Hang them from a mirror, or attach them to a frame or create a full wall feature!

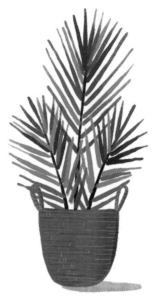

PALMS

Let's start with this simple but confusing fact: palms are not trees. Yes, every Florida or California resort is lined with those tall trunks crowned by waving fronds that everyone calls palm trees, but they are actually a kind of flowering plant. Not that it really matters when you're looking for a plant to grow inside, but hopefully you find it reassuring that you need not expect your small potted palm to produce enough coconuts for *Gilligan's Island*.

Palms are a wonderful embellishment for your interior design, since they evoke soothing tropical beach vacations, adding a lush, sun-soaked feel to the darkest and coldest of winter days. In general, they like what we like—warm temperatures, moderate light, and a pleasant level of humidity—but different palm species will want slightly different arrangements, so make sure to match your palm selection to your space. Areca palms or parlor palms are good starters. Crown palms and sago palms make for a more striking look (but watch out for sago palms if you have pets! They're extremely poisonous. More on that in chapter 2). Now turn on an ocean wave sound machine, and you and your palm can both relax.

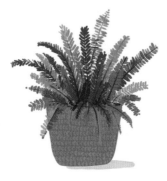

FERNS

The biggest challenge in bringing a new fern into your home is deciding which of the more than twelve thousand different types is the right one for you! As one of earth's oldest plant varieties (there are fern fossils as old as three hundred million years), they have had plenty of time to develop some individuality. Pick a fern that likes the kind of light you can provide and the level of care you want to invest. A Boston fern may only need an occasional check-in, but that dramatic staghorn fern will need a steady parental hand to guide it.

Most ferns like moist soil to grow—that's why you'll find them unfurling fronds with such abandon in the spring. To re-create this mood at home, set a fern pot in a tray filled with pebbles and water. The water will slowly evaporate and your fern will enthusiastically suck up that damper air.

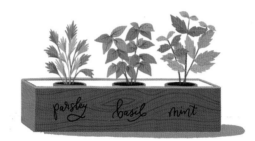

Edibles

This isn't a tough one to explain. These are the plants you can eat—like herbs, aloe, flowers, even fruits and vegetables. If you are an energetic cook, you will love having fresh herbs readily on hand to add to your meal. Picture fresh basil leaves torn over pasta, fragrant chives minced into omelets, nasturtium flowers tossed into salads. Even if you and cooking do not go together, pots of rosemary or lavender make for beautiful and aromatic windowsill decor.

For the ambitious indoor vegetable gardener, larger pots or hydroponic towers can produce lovely fresh fruits and vegetables, but these will take a lot of care and attention, not to mention the necessity of playing the part of a bee for fertilization. Consider whether that's the kind of relationship you're looking for with your houseplant.

One thing to keep in mind is that most herbs and other edibles require lots of sunshine. Sunny windowsills and doorways make good homes for edibles. If your indoor growing space lacks large amounts of bright light, you might want to try another option.

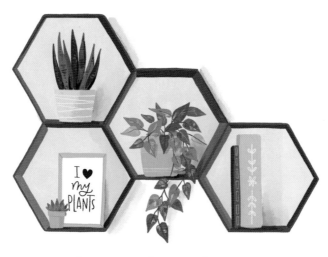

Putting Down Roots

If you haven't been scared off plant parenthood by this list of plants and their needs, then let's move on to the next level in making sure you're fully prepared for the ramifications of flora/fauna cohabitation. Can you commit?

The first step is to think about who else lives in your home. If you're solo, you get to design your space as you see fit. If that means air plants tucked into your shower caddy and pothos vines draped down your bookshelves, go for it! Let your plant family express you.

The upside and downside of sharing your home with pets or people is that while they may share in your joy of growing your own indoor garden, they also will probably want a say. Cats especially like a lot of input on what kind of plants appear in the home and how they will be displayed. A hanging spider plant with dangling tendrils is a terrible feline temptation for attack. And cats, dogs, and toddlers need to be protected from snacking on plants that may be beautiful but poisonous if ingested.

Another consideration is how much time you want to invest in this new addition. If you're still working out how to care for yourself, it might be a good idea to start with one of the more indestructible species (looking at you, cast-iron plant). If you have that needy urge to nurture that irritates your friends, your partner, your coworkers, your pets, or your grown children, you might put your energy toward a delicate bloomer that needs regular maintenance.

Take a look at your schedule. If you travel a lot for work or fun, make sure you have a plant that needs only occasional watering and attendance. If you work from home, a forest of greenery may be just what you need to keep you focused and productive.

Mary Beth Shaddix, plant writer and owner of Maple Valley Nursery near Birmingham, Alabama, says, "Houseplants take a different amount of time and attention. Indoors it doesn't get rain or sunshine on a regular basis. A houseplant is completely dependent on you."

Houseplants are so much more than an artistic adornment like a throw pillow. Introducing this separate but similar life-form into our homes and work spaces can bring us better health—better air and better modes of thought. Bringing plant life into your home life can be a boost to your sense of well-being.

Plants can also tie us to our past, a living memory of fleeting vacations or the deeper connections to childhood memories of plants our parents and grandparents grew inside and outside. The plant that you use to decorate your home can tell a story. Add that extra depth to your life's root structure and select a plant that evokes something of you:

- an on-trend, in-the-moment, grammable zebra plant with artistic leaves so neatly put together, they can look unreal
- a brilliantly colored but fickle orchid that blooms only once a year
- a rampant tangle of mint that bursts its pot and produces leaves for more mojitos than you can possibly (or safely) consume
- a wild, tropical bird of paradise conjuring images of exotic getaways and warm weather
- a traditional Norfolk Island pine, its feathered fronds calling to mind northern forests, Christmas trees, and winter celebrations (though in fact it hails from the South Pacific!)

Or pick them all and cultivate a jungle of indoor houseplant possibilities.

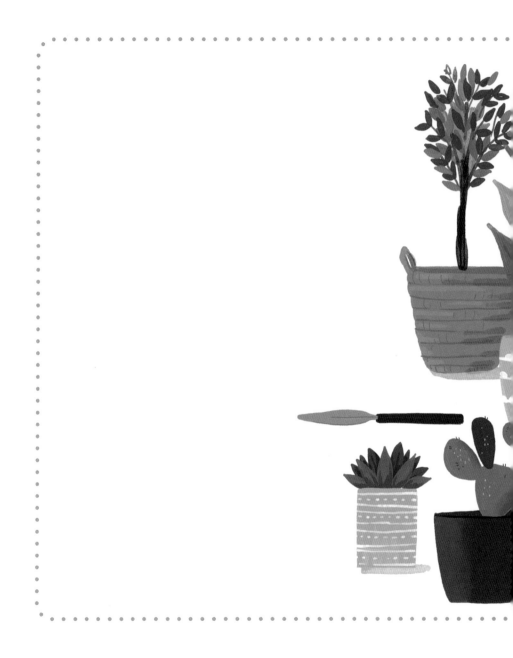

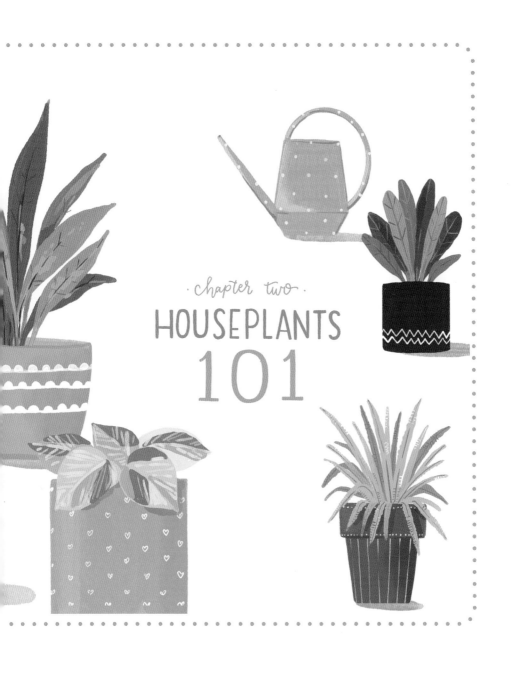

chapter two

HOUSEPLANTS
101

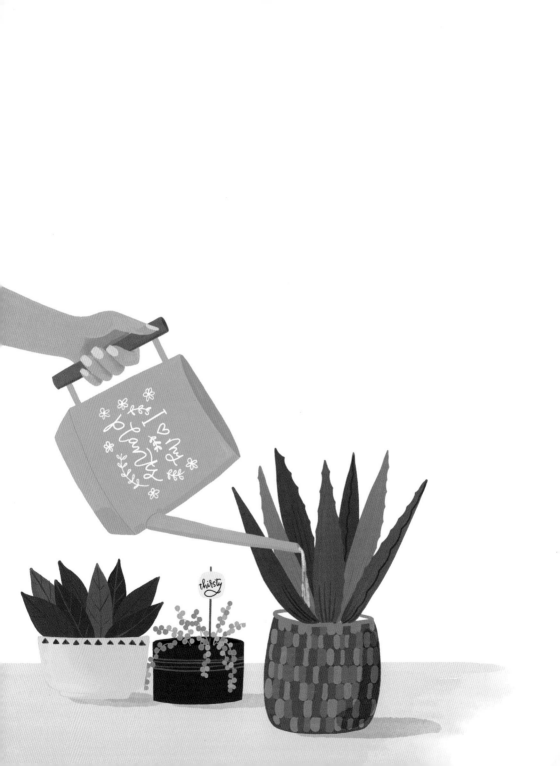

wning a houseplant is not the hardest work you will ever have to do. In fact, most of the time, it really can't be called work. This is one of those relationships you just relax into and enjoy. Your plant is never annoyed you didn't text back right away, never forgets (well, or remembers) your birthday, and rarely burdens you with its emotional problems.

Even so, it can't be completely ignored! While some plants are higher maintenance than others, each is a living being that does need occasional TLC. Identifying how much of your attention your plant needs is the beginning of a beautiful relationship.

Ryan and Meriel Lesseig of Air Plant Design Studio present us with this clear formula: "A plant's care breaks down to these important principles: light, air, and water."

Let's start with water.

WATERING

You knew this section was coming. Like us, plants are made of mostly water and need to consume water just as much as their human companions. It's essential. What they don't need is the eight glasses a day that doctors inflict on humans.

The basic rule of thumb for plant-watering schedules is actually a rule of finger. Stick your finger into the soil or moss around your plant. Is it damp? Your plant is probably fine. Is it wet? Lay off the water—we don't want to drown it! Is it bone dry? *Water. Stat!*

Part of what puts a plant on "easy plants for first-time plant owners" lists is that the watering process is undemanding. As your thumb gets greener, taking on needier plants can be rewarding, but make sure you are ready to launch into helicopter plant parenting first.

Overwatering is just as much of a risk to a plant as forgetting to water. Watering is not an everyday thing unless you are raising a water lily. Plants like marinating in a bath about as much as your cat. "A customer asked me which plant to buy that could take being watered every day because she needed to be needed by *someone* or *something*. Most indoor foliage will die if watered every day," says Joyce Mast, "Plant Mom" at Bloomscape, a Detroit-based online plant delivery service.

Each plant will require a different amount of water, but develop a schedule or habit for water checks and it can become a part of your routine—and maybe even a project you enjoy. Many indoor-plant owners make watering a ritual. Once a week or every other week, they'll round up any plant that looks thirsty and collect them in a sink or bathtub to get them all watered—and carefully drained—at once.

"The simplest thing to remember is that plants are not pets! You can give a dog as much water as you want, but they'll decide when it's enough and stop drinking. Plants can't, and they will drown," says Matt Kostelnick, senior horticulturist at indoor office plant company Ambius. Enough water for most plants will mean filling the pot gently until water is coming out of the drainage holes, then stopping.

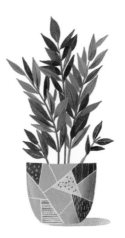

HOW TO WATER YOUR ZZ PLANT

ZZ plants ("ZZ" is a nickname from the proper Latin nomenclature, *Zamioculcas zamiifolia*—try saying that five times fast), with their shiny, zigzagged leaves, are both striking to look at and easy to please when it comes to watering. They want you to forget to water and don't get their feelings hurt by neglect. Let the soil completely dry out and then water thoroughly, enough for it to flow freely through the soil and out the pot's drainage holes. This will ensure that your plant is wet, the soil is wet, and

Drain it! We can't say this enough: your pot must, must, *must* allow water to flow out. Standing water at the bottom of your pot causes root rot.

the excess water has washed away any soil or fertilizer impurities. Now just wait for it to dry out again—check in a couple of weeks.

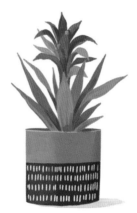

HOW TO WATER YOUR BROMELIAD

Bromeliads, like ZZ plants, are cool with a little drought. Water thoroughly once a week or less, then let the soil dry out. You do need to pay a little more attention to checking the bromeliads' drainage. Bromeliads cannot sit in water—their roots will rot if constantly wet and kill your plant from the bottom up. Pot them in a container and soil that drain thoroughly, so they can't soak. While their roots don't like the wet, their leaves do. Bromeliads hail from the tropics; they like humidity! If your indoor climate can't provide humid air (this will be an issue especially in cold-climate winter months when heaters pump out dry air), you can create a little private humidity just for your very own tropical plant: set its pot in a tray of wet gravel. The water in the gravel will evaporate and your bromeliad can enjoy that damper air.

How to Water Your Staghorn Fern

There is a certain amount of trial and error in perfectly watering a staghorn fern, and usually more than one method will be necessary. These are epiphytes, like air plants, so they aren't grown in a pot of soil that you can test for dampness but are attached to a plaque, hanging basket, or wall mount. A staghorn fern should never dry out completely like your ZZ plant. It likes humidity, so locate this kind of plant in a damp environment—like the bathroom, where you take steamy showers—or be prepared to mist it with a spray bottle periodically. Sometimes it will need a heavier watering, perhaps once a week. Spray it down thoroughly, focusing on the base, not the leaves, in a shower or sink, and then let it drip dry before you rehang it. It's also a good idea to wipe any moisture off the leaves to avoid fungus growth.

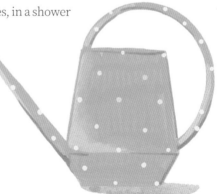

How to Water Your Venus Fly Trap

This is a popular gift for a kid because they're a little creepy (a carnivorous plant? Ew). Usually they die as quickly as they're acquired because 1) kids and 2) they are picky about water. They turn up their toothy leaves at tap water; give them distilled water or fresh rainwater only.

Potting

Perhaps you brought your first plant home in a cute little pot that complements your home decor. Great! You're all set. But is your plant? Does your plant even like its new home? Did you even ask? Your plant would be the first to tell you that a good pot ought to be more than pleasing to the eye. It must answer your plant's needs, not just your aesthetic.

No matter what they say, in this case, size matters. Get the right size pot for your plant. An orchid or bromeliad likes to be "underpotted" in a pot that fits its roots snugly. If it's set in too large a pot, it will focus on growing lots of roots, not lots of foliage or flowers. Most other plants get stressed at being underpotted, their leaves becoming limp, their roots forcing through the bottom of the pot, desperately searching for new growing space. But "overpotting" will bother them, too—a little indoor plant in a huge pot will yellow and even lose its leaves. Its small roots can't reach the huge quantities of water the soil in the large pot is soaking up,

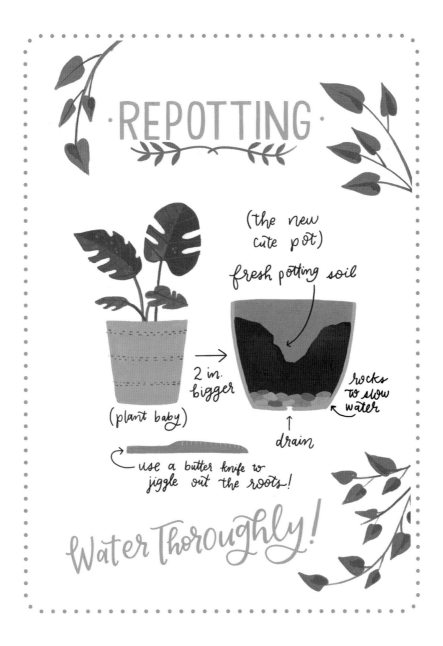

· REPOTTING ·

(the new cute pot)

fresh potting soil

2 in. bigger

(plant baby)

rocks to slow water

drain

use a butter knife to jiggle out the roots!

Water Thoroughly!

so the water just collects in a muddy mess at the bottom of the pot and the roots rot in that dense muck. Your pot should easily fit the root ball of your plant, with about two inches of new-growth space around it.

Pot prepared, now start your soil. Don't overthink this. Most plants just need regular potting soil. Potting mixes are usually already fertilized and aerated to give your plant its best growing start. But you really will need the potting soil, not just whatever dirt you have handy, according to Julie Bawden-Davis, master gardener and founder of HealthyHouseplants .com. "People will go outside and dig up dirt from the garden. It's not the right consistency for indoor growing—it's way too heavy! Roots need to be able to move around in there. The thing to remember is that what's going on in the pot is all that plant has to work with."

There will come a time when you need to repot. Don't worry! This means you're doing a good job and your plant is very happy and growing well in your home. It has simply outgrown its old clothes and tired out its soil. Give it a little bit bigger quarters and some delicious mineral-rich new dirt and it will thrive.

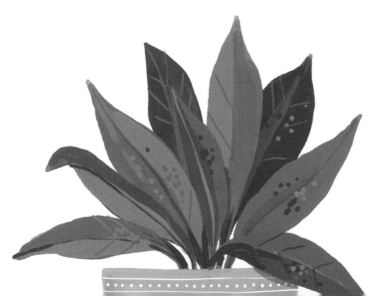

Don't Forget the Drainage!

If you like the size, now check that you like the drip. Like a baby, a plant doesn't like to sit in a wet diaper. Make sure your plant's pot has good drainage. That means a hole in the bottom of the pot. When you water, you need water to drip through the soil and flow into a tray or sink, not pool around your plant's roots. As mentioned previously, soaking roots can lead to rotting roots, and that spells the end for your plant.

Still, many plants are sold in holeless pots. These may look nice in the store, but they won't work for plant longevity. If your pot doesn't have a hole in the bottom, find one that does. Can't part with that adorable pot? If you're the handy-around-the-house type, you can drill holes in the pot's base. Those of us with less drill savvy should look into a pot insert—repot your plant into a plastic pot (with drainage holes!) and slip the whole thing into the decorative pot. To water, take out the pot insert, water the plant, drain, and return the insert to its attractive outerwear.

How to Repot a *Monstera deliciosa*

The baby *Monstera deliciosa* plant has solid, heart-shaped leaves. The teen-aged plant's leaves begin to part into fingers. The mature plant's leaves add oval perforations between the fingers like a crocheted doily. These lacy, tropical beauties grow enthusiastically and only get better looking as they age, so please just give them the opportunity by repotting as they grow.

1. Get the new pot ready—it shouldn't be more than two inches larger in diameter than the old pot. Fill it with fresh potting mix, leaving space for the plant. Don't overfill it with dirt; you want some room at the top for water to collect. If you're worried about soil washing through a large drainage hole when you water, you can scatter broken pot shards or small rocks in the bottom before adding the soil to slow the flow.

2. Slide the plant out of the existing pot. Sometimes tipping it on its side and using a knife or thin spatula will help it jiggle out with its roots mostly intact. If the roots are particularly densely packed, use your fingers to loosen them up a bit.

3. Set the plant in the new pot and fill in the space around the roots with fresh soil. Gently press it into place to get rid of air pockets.

4. Water thoroughly to let the old plant and new soil settle in together.

5. *Monsteras* like to climb, so repotting time is also a good time to add a trellis or stake to your pot.

How to Repot a Cactus

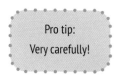

Pro tip:
Very carefully!

If you're potting cacti or succulents, this is the time to select a specialty potting mix to help water drain faster for these dry-climate plants. Something sandy, with perlite or vermiculite—maybe something labeled "cactus potting soil"?

1. You know the drill: get the pot ready. The new pot should only be about an inch larger in diameter than the existing one, because cacti grow slowly and need *really* good water drainage. Fill it about halfway with that fancy soil.

2. This is where it gets interesting. Wear gloves. Wrap newspaper or magazine pages around the cactus to protect your hands as you carefully remove it from the old pot.

3. Using that protective paper, place the cactus in the new pot and add soil around it—maybe use a spoon or other tool when adding soil so your fingers don't get too close to the prickles.

4. Water it well, but then leave it alone to dry out completely before you water again. Desert plant, remember?

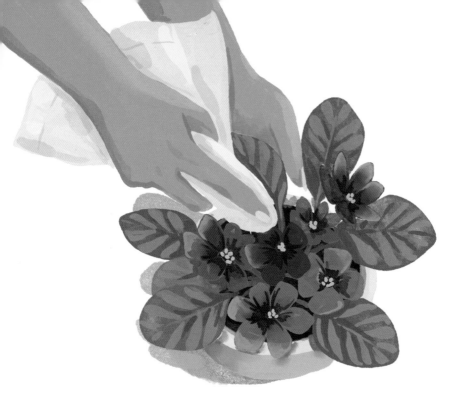

DUSTING

This is more than tidying up; this is to help your plant breathe. Like a Bond girl covered in gold paint, a plant covered with dust suffocates. As dust builds up on leaves, it blocks the sunlight, making it harder for your plant to photosynthesize. Photosynthesis is the plant's version of eating—plants use sunlight to turn carbon dioxide (reminder: this is what you breathe out) into sugars that they use for energy, or food. If the sunlight can't get through the layer of filth graying those leaves, that plant will not eat tonight.

There isn't a set time frame for how often plants need to be dusted. It will depend on your location. Homes near interstates, congested highways, or dirt roads are going to be dustier. Check your plant for buildup and clean it when the dust is too heavy to blow away.

When we're talking about dusting, please put away the Lysol and the furniture polish. This is not the place for chemicals. Damp cloths, a bathtub, or a duster will do the job best.

How to Dust Your Fiddle-Leaf Fig Tree

Larger, sturdy, smooth-leaved plants like a fiddle-leaf fig tree or a ZZ plant can be dusted just as you would dust your coffee table. Dampen a washcloth with water and gently wipe down the leaves. Or spray each leaf with water and wipe it clean. If it's really grimy, you can use a few drops of soap in the water, but be sure to wipe off the soap, too! If you use soap, protect the plant's roots by covering them with a towel or plastic wrap while you rinse. If this sounds time-consuming, it is. But it's not something you have to do every day unless you live next to a gravel pit.

How to Dust Your Areca Palm

If you had to individually wipe each frond on a luxuriant palm, you would go nuts. Instead, place this kind of plant in a bathtub or sink and rinse it down with a shower or sprayer. This is a quick job! Let the leaves dry thoroughly afterward so they don't develop a fungus, but since you're not using soap this time, the roots will be perfectly happy with a little extra water.

How to Dust Your African Violet

Plants with fuzzy or delicate leaves won't take well to a bath or a wipe down. Time to break out that feather (or synthetic) duster! A mushroom brush will also work to gently clean the leaves. For that matter, a moustache brush would probably do as well.

Plant Panics

There are times when you come home to a drooping, yellow-leaved plant or spider mites crawling through your croton. Don't panic by throwing out that plant. Go through this checklist to see if it can be saved:

1. When was the last time you watered your plant? If it looks limp and the soil is as dry as a martini, just apologize and get it wet.
2. You've been watering every day? Just stop! Give it some space and let it dry out. Check the roots to verify they're not waterlogged and rotting.
3. Yellow, droopy, sad, and filthy. If you looked like this, you'd take a shower. Doesn't your plant deserve a rinse or dust off, too?

4. Roots are squeezing through drainage holes and your plant looks exhausted? Bust it out of jail and repot.

5. Fertilizing is to a plant what a midafternoon snack is to you. It just needs a little pick-me-up every few months. When newly potted, that fresh soil is full of good nutrition for your hungry plant, but as months go by, the plant has sucked out all the good stuff and the soil needs replenishing. Pick a liquid or, even better, a slow-release fertilizer and follow instructions on how often to use—it varies by brand and plant.

6. Patchy, blotchy leaves? It's not a bad complexion—it's probably just a fungus. Whether coming from air or soil, a fungus will take over your plant, and fast. Catch it early and treat with an antifungal spray. Or, since these sprays can be toxic to pets and people, try a baking soda solution—a teaspoon of powder to a quart of water—sprayed on the damaged leaves.

7. Spider mites, mealy bugs, scales, aphids, oh my. If you spot these little vampires sucking plant juices uninvited, get rid of them right away. Spray spider mites and aphids with insecticidal soap or neem oil on repeat until the bugs are gone. Cut and toss leaves and branches infected with mealy bugs and scales, or wipe them off with a rag or cotton ball soaked in rubbing alcohol. These pests can be hard to eradicate,

so be sure to isolate the affected plant until they are gone, and keep a close eye on any other plants to prevent spreading.

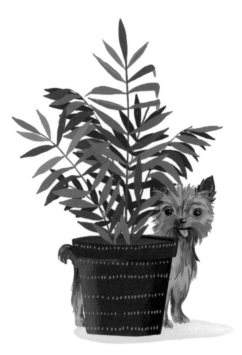

Pets Do Not Have Green Paws

Now that you are prepared to defend your plant from insect pests, let's talk about the other pests in your house: pets and kids.

If you don't have either, skip ahead to the next section, but keep these tips in mind should you ever risk it all on bringing additional life-forms into your plant's home.

Of course any animal can coexist peacefully with plant life—we grew up together, after all. If you are introducing a new plant into a dog's or cat's habitat, however, you'll want to make sure they are compatible.

First, there is the issue of safety. Pets test out a new acquaintance by putting it in their mouths, whether it's a new person or a new sofa or an interesting-looking electrical cord. Any plant, if enough is ingested, will make a dog or cat sick, but some plants are flat-out deadly. If your pet shares its home with you, make sure to check which plants are poisonous to your pet before bringing them home. Popular plants like peace lilies, aloe vera, pothos, and even the ZZ plant and fiddle-leaf fig trees mentioned previously will not be good choices. Some safer alternatives could include spider plants, peperomia, haworthia, and *some* palm species.

The fastest and easiest source on plant toxicity is the ASPCA website (aspca.org). Search the organization's extensive list of toxic and nontoxic plants by pet species both for ideas for safe plants and to verify that your preferred plant isn't a pet killer.

The second issue is whether you can persuade your pets not to destroy that gorgeous and lovingly chosen nonpoisonous new plant. Cats adore knocking objects off tables and dogs find it so exciting to jump on and chew up any home furnishings (not to mention the possibility of a truly undesirable fire hydrant confusion).

One option is to position your plants in locations not easily accessed by pets. A high table or hanging a plant puts the temptation out of reach for most dogs, though unfortunately the same can't be said for a cat. Cascading vines are too much of a temptation for a vigorous leap, pull, crash.

Never Put a Cactus in the Bathroom

Hang plants out of their reach or in a location that doesn't attract their attention. A plant big enough that they can't knock it over could work, if you don't mind finding kitty climbing your banana palm.

Training can be helpful, too. Spray a nasty-tasting formula (there are several "flavors" at pet stores—find the one your pet hates the most) on plants repeatedly for a few weeks or place lemon rinds in the soil, as most cats can't stand the smell. Pairing the spray with distraction can also be effective. Try giving your cat its very own plant to care for and hope that it might be less interested in yours. How about a little wheatgrass or catnip for kitty to nibble?

These same concerns apply to small children, a species similarly given to putting things in their mouths indiscriminately. Every Christmas, emergency rooms get visited by kids who thought the pretty yellow "candies" growing on the holiday poinsettia would be good to eat. And any parent will tell you: if you think you have successfully hidden something from your toddler, turn your back and wait five minutes.

Stick to nontoxic plants when you have little ones. It may seem like forever right now, but someday they'll be old enough to know not to nibble that sago palm before you have to repot your *Monstera*.

Fun Facts

Now that you are a proud plant owner, you will be anxious to share your newfound enthusiasm and knowledge. Here are some random and entertaining plant tidbits to enliven your cocktail party conversation:

- Bamboo can grow thirty-five inches in a single day.
- In the 1600s, Dutch merchants were so into tulips that they were extremely valuable—until that obsession crashed Holland's whole economy.
- Corpse flowers stink like death to attract flies for pollination.
- While we humans eat or use more than two thousand different varieties of plants, we should probably watch our backs—there are more than six hundred kinds of carnivorous plants, including one that can consume a rat!
- But don't worry, 85 percent of plant life is in the ocean.
- Caffeine may get you moving in the morning, but for a coffee plant, it's a natural pesticide.
- Vanilla pods grow on orchids.
- Saffron comes from the stamen of a crocus.
- The Australian suicide plant has a sting so incredibly painful and lasting (years!) that people have killed themselves after touching it.
- Whatever direction a seed is dropped into the ground, its sprout can always find its way up to the sun. Would that we could all follow its example.

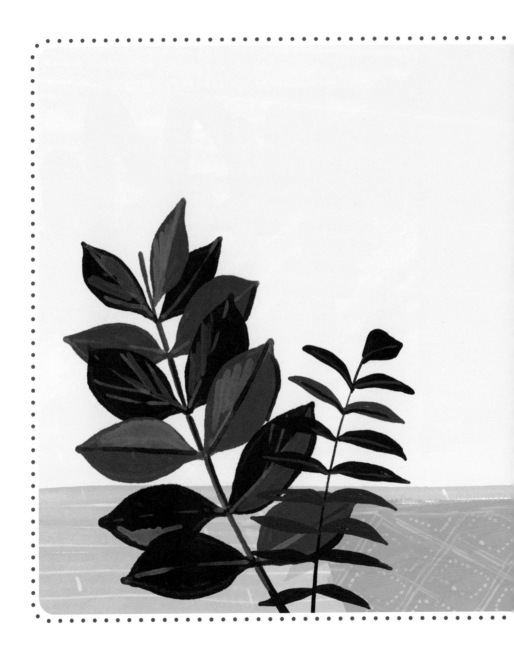

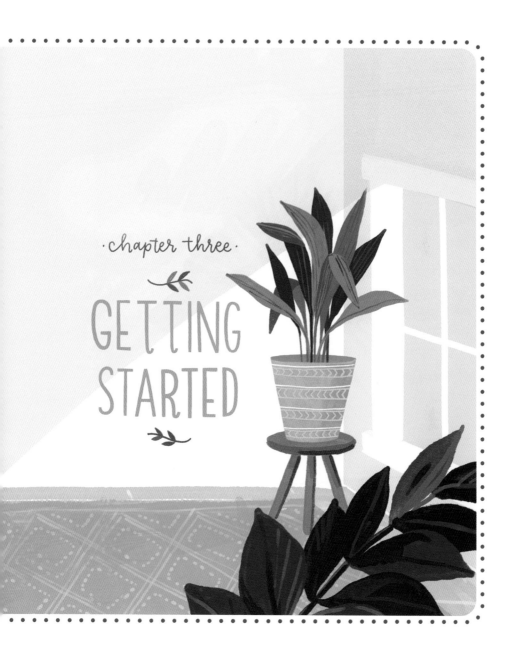

· chapter three ·

GETTING STARTED

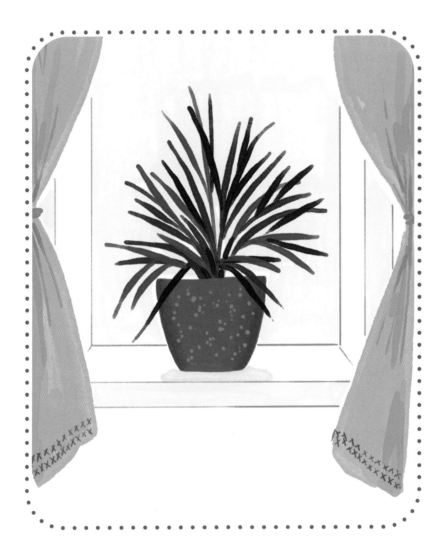

Having read the first two chapters, you now know just enough to be dangerous. You have ambitious visions of rare succulents nestled on your bedroom windowsill, exotic and impossible-to-find orchids lining your bookshelves, and festoons of hanging plants in every corner from the kitchen to the dining room. But let's be honest—you're still rooted to the sofa, binge-watching TV because you're secretly really nervous about which plant to make your first victim, er, guest. Don't be scared. We'll take this slowly.

There are some solid, easy plants to suggest for beginners, but let's start with *you*. What kind of home are you prepared to offer a plant?

Let There Be Light

All those useful labels pasted to plant pots at the garden store say things like "bright indirect light" or "low light." What on this green earth does that mean?

The first step in choosing the best plants for your living space is to identify the natural light sources in your home. Translation? Find the windows.

Next, you'll want to know which directions the windows face. South-facing windows get more intense, or direct, light. North-facing windows get less intense light, or indirect light—if the window is otherwise unobstructed, the light can still be "bright" while also being indirect. East- and west-facing windows tend to get medium light. What is medium light, you ask? Stand by your east/west windows. It's that.

Now, what kind of view do you enjoy? If you're looking out at shady trees (yay!) or the wall of another building (sigh), this window probably doesn't get a huge amount of bright sun. This means it's "low light." If you can't determine from your view how long the sun will come through your window, you should refer to this general guide, though it may involve a lot of time sitting and staring at a window:

- Low light: less than four hours of sun
- Medium light: four to six hours of sun
- Bright light: more than six hours of sun

A couple of other light tips: Rotating your plant periodically will keep it evenly leaved and growing straight—the plant will lean into the sun. The brighter the light, the faster water will evaporate from the soil and from the plant itself, so consider the quality of light while learning your watering schedule.

Whatever light you have, you can still grow a plant. Just choose wisely.

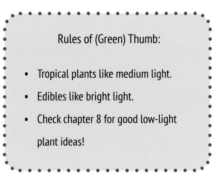

Rules of (Green) Thumb:

- Tropical plants like medium light.
- Edibles like bright light.
- Check chapter 8 for good low-light plant ideas!

A Plant to Grow On

Before you get intimidated by the rows of plant possibilities at your local garden shop, consider some options that the greatest plant experts in the world and even the biggest houseplant-growing failures will admit are foolproof. Or at least nearly foolproof.

Cast-Iron Plant

Also called a barroom plant or an aspidistra, or *Aspidistra elatior* when it's feeling Latin, it is nicknamed "cast iron" because it is as hard to destroy as a cast-iron pan. It can grow outside. It can grow inside. It can grow in very dim light. It can deal when you forget to water for a month. It doesn't mind getting cold. It doesn't mind being hot. Insects avoid it. Full, leafy, and charming, this plant is ready for whatever you throw at it. Now if only you could find a significant other with the same qualities. . . .

Originally from the northern East Asian islands and Japan, the cast-iron plant made its way to Europe more than two hundred years ago as a popular if somewhat bourgeois parlor plant. Picture it taking its place in Victorian society, inhabiting the spiderwebbed corners of Miss Havisham's dining room and surviving a thoughtless Sherlock Holmes long enough for Mrs. Hudson to take pity on it. Less refined aspidistras could be found in barroom corners in the stultifying atmosphere, breathing the toxic gas lamp, coal fire, and cigar fumes, maybe squatting next to the spittoon, back to the wall.

If it can survive all that, it can survive you.

The cast-iron plant's leaves are long dark-green sheaths, about four inches wide and two feet long. It's part of the lily family of plants and it can sometimes flower, tiny purple flowers that cluster near the soil—but don't grow it for its bloom. Its charm is its steadfast greenery.

Set your cast-iron plant in a well-draining pot and position it to cheer an otherwise gloomy corner. Whatever you do, don't put it in bright sunshine. Its leaves will burn and no amount of aloe vera (even homegrown) will soothe dry, brown aspidistra leaves.

It definitely needs watering—it's a plant—but it can survive a month or so without it. Dim lighting means lower evaporation, and this plant likes to keep its roots on the dry side. Before you water, test the soil for any dampness, about an inch or two below the surface. Dust off the leaves once a year (or more often if you picked a particularly dusty corner), fertilize annually as well, and that plant is ready to go. It grows slowly, so you probably won't have to repot very often—sometimes going as long as four or five years! It's ready for a new pot when its roots grow out of the pot. With a little care, it can grow as high as two feet and live a long time.

Now that you love your carefree cast iron, don't you want more? You're in luck—this is a "rhizomatous" plant, which means it will create new little cast-iron plants for you from its own rootstock. The plant's primary stems, or rhizomes, will send out horizontal subsidiary stems under the soil. When one of these side-piece rhizomes grows its stem above the soil and produces at least two small leaves, it's ready for harvesting. Break off that section of new rhizome with the leaves on it and pot it, keeping it uncharacteristically moist and warm until new shoots form. Now you've got a new cast-iron plant!

If by this time you feel that the cast-iron plant is your perfect match, check out the alternative varieties of the species to change things up: variegated green-and-white okame, white-tipped asahi, or Lennon's song, with yellow vertical stripes.

If, however, you feel the cast-iron plant serves as too unpleasant a reminder of repressive Victorian respectability and classism, first put down the George Orwell, then take a look at a less tradition-bound alternative, like the ubiquitous pothos.

POTHOS

Pothos is a plant with a bit of an identity crisis.

Pothos is a genus of flowering, vining tropical plants. There are tons of varieties, though not often found as houseplants. What most stores are selling under this name is actually *Epipremnum aureum,* in a completely different genus. It's commonly called golden pothos, aka devil's ivy, Ceylon creeper, money plant, etc. It was once an immigrant from Mo'orea in the French Polynesia Society Islands, but is now a resident of any and all tropical and subtropical ecosystems.

Its name problem derives from botantists' habit of naming plants by observable features, not genetic makeup. But golden pothos got its name well before complex genetic testing was available, so we'll give those old botantists a pass.

Less excusable is plant stores confusing the labels of pothos and phil-odendron. More on that later.

But what's in a name anyway? A pothos by any other name is still a lively addition to your home, and so easy to grow that it has earned a reputation as an invasive species in tropical climates, where when planted outside it can take over a garden and climb up trees, producing leaves as large as dinner plates. Even in more temperate locales, you've probably spotted it filling built-in planters in indoor malls.

Pothos is a vine, with green heart-shaped leaves usually dashed with a little color, yellow or white. When maintained well, it will form a nice bushy plant with trailing vines. It lasts a long time.

Like the cast-iron plant, pothos prefers a little neglect. It likes bright, indirect light, in that four-to-six-hour range, but won't tolerate much direct light. It likes damp but not wet soil, so it needs to dry out well between waterings. Add fertilizer monthly, since potting soil has few nutrients. Dusting is easy—rinse it off in a shower. For the first-time house-planter, pothos is helpful because it's such a good communicator. Just learn its language:

- Droopy leaves = too dry
- Black spots = too wet
- Pale leaves = too much sun
- All-green leaves (no variegation) = not enough sun
- Brown leaves = too much dry air

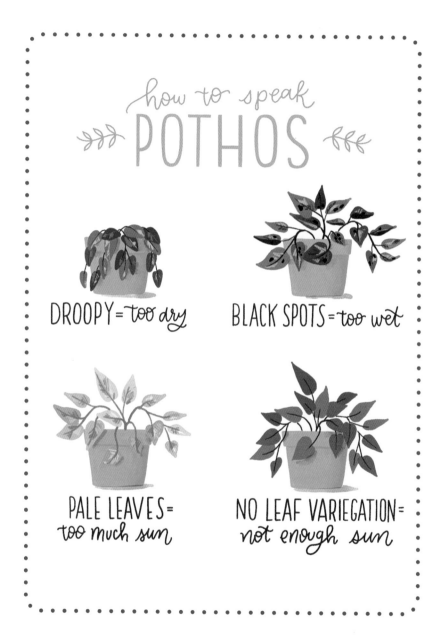

Getting pothos to grow in the shape you want will require you to take the conversational upper hand, however. You decide its shape as it grows. If your pothos is looking leggy, prune back its trailing stems and the plant will be bushier and more compact. Just cut the vine about a quarter inch above a leaf. You can even use discarded trimmings to propagate new plants! If you like a cascading look, try directing the vines up a trellis or draping down a bookshelf. Prune extraneous and secondary stems so those dominant stems can really grow.

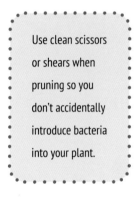

Use clean scissors or shears when pruning so you don't accidentally introduce bacteria into your plant.

There are some fantastic varieties of pothos, so you can match your vine to your style. Try white-and-green-patterned Marble Queen to give your room a classic look, or the outrageous Neon with brilliant chartreuse leaves, or dainty Pearls and Jade, almost as pretty as its name.

The downside of pothos is that it is highly toxic to pets. If kitty takes a nibble, kitty will be taking a trip to the vet. So if you have the type of pet that takes an interest in your new houseplant hobby, place this one out of reach. It is also toxic to humans, so (we don't really have to say this, do we?) don't eat it.

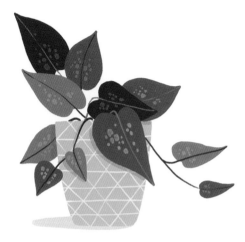

Philodendron

Philodendrons and pothos, when grown indoors, look so similar at a passing glance that getting upset at someone calling your plant by the wrong name is kind of like getting upset at someone not knowing the difference between your two goldfish, Fin and Goldie.

That said, garden centers should know better. And here's how *you* tell:

- Philodendron leaves are truly heart shaped, with a wide curve spreading out from the stem. Pothos have a narrower, more oval shape sloping downward from the stem.
- Both plants produce aerial roots from their trailing vines. Philodendron roots are thin, yellow, and wispy. Pothos roots are little dark knobs.

- Take a close look at the spot where the leaf connects to the vine. The leaf stem, or petiole, is round and fleshy on a philodendron, whereas a pothos petiole tapers and curves to clasp the vine.
- Where the philodendron leaf stem meets the vine, it will produce a sheath that turns brown and papery as it ages. This is unique to the philodendron, and not to be found on a pothos vine.
- Philodendrons are South American, and pothos are from the South Pacific. This may or may not come up in conversation.
- The name "philodendron" comes from Greek words for love and tree. In Greek mythology, Pothos hung out with Aphrodite, goddess of love, and symbolized yearning.

Now that you are a philodendron vs. pothos expert, here's one more thing to remember: it really doesn't matter that much. You care for each plant in the same way: give it light, but keep it out of direct sun; water only when the top inch or so of soil is dry; "dust" with a little shower; fertilize monthly to urge on bigger, more mature leaves; repot annually. Some varieties tend to be smaller and bushier, but most popularly sold types will grow into long, trailing vines that you can train to frame your room in that untamed jungle look.

Which you like better—philodendron or pothos—is a personal choice.

Or possibly a "what's available at the plant store on that day you decide you simply can't live any longer without a tropical vine enhancing your windowsill" choice.

Spider Plant

We're on a roll with these tropical trailers. Let's keep it going in the same vine.

You've definitely seen a spider plant (also called airplane plant and chlorophytum) before—its narrow, leggy, green-and-yellow leaves bending out from a bushy cluster that looks so . . . arachnid. These are some of the most popular indoor plants. In the seventies, if you didn't have a spider plant hanging from a macrame pot hanger over the TV, we're pretty sure you were disqualified from the disco on Saturday night.

Spider plants were originally found in Africa and arrived in European and American drawing rooms in the nineteenth century. (Those Victorians and their houseplants! But hey, if they could keep them alive in all that coal-fire-black air, surely you can keep one alive in your cozy den.) Their popularity trended upward again in the 1970s, a peak period for indoor plants in general, coming in hot from the 1960s' flower power with the founding of Earth Day in 1970. Check any popular disco-era TV show and you'll find a houseplant in the background decor.

One cute thing about that iconic seventies spider plant is that it propagates so easily and lasts so long that you can probably call your grandmother or that one weird aunt for a cutting of her spider plant and keep it all in the family.

As you would expect of such a groovy plant, they are pretty chill about how much light they need, though their leaves will turn brown in too much direct sun. Water them well when their soil is dry—they like a fast-drying potting mix so their roots don't soak, but they will need extra water in the summer months. They don't need to be repotted often because they work harder at making babies than at growing roots—who can blame them?—so only move to a larger pot when the root ball starts growing through or over the pot.

If you care for your spider plant well, you will get spider babies! This may sound a little like bringing home a hamster from the pet store and discovering it's pregnant, but spider-plant free love is nothing to be scared of. It can create a whole family of houseplants to decorate your home and share with your bemused friends. The parent plant produces lovely little white flowers, which grow on trailing yellow stems; from each of these, a small spider plantlet grows. Wait until the tiny plant starts growing aerial roots, clip it from the stem, and pot it (or, if it has yet to develop roots, let it sit in water for a few weeks and roots will grow). Brand-new spider plant, at your service.

Spider plants truly are here to serve. They are not toxic for cats and dogs and even humans who like to chew houseplants. They are also especially good at removing toxins, sucking in formaldehyde from your dirty indoor air.

Love your spider plant like your spider plant loves you. And peace, man.

Peace Lily

Finally, a flowering plant to make you feel like an accomplished houseplant owner without really any more effort than any of the tropical vines require. The peace lily, and its cousin the calla lily, aren't closely related to the heavy-scented, pollen-laden blooms of summer gardens. This is a year-round companion to breathe fresh air into even your dark winter months.

The peace lily produces a dense cluster of dark-green, shiny oval leaves and can grow up to three or four feet tall—it's one that can be used as a floor plant or kept smaller on tables and desks. It produces long-lasting white flowers consisting of a hoodlike sheath offsetting a more off-white center stalk.

A tropical rain forest native, it likes its water but will let you know when it's ready—droopy leaves mean it's time to water. Those leaves will perk right back up with a good drink! A medium amount of light and a good wipe-off to remove dust periodically will keep it happy. There are lots of varieties of the peace lily, so you can pick the mature plant size that suits you, from the "power petite" variety to the strikingly named "Mauna Loa supreme."

Sadly, though, this peace comes with a little poison—it is another one poisonous to your pets. The upside is that it's another one on NASA's list of air-purifying plants to make each deep breath a more peaceful experience.

Plant Proficiency

As a careful reader, you have no doubt noticed by now some themes and common features among all these "easy" plants: low light is okay, don't overwater, repot annually at most, drainage matters. This is a more concise and doable list than, say, following the directions on how to build that Ikea bookshelf from which your pothos (or is it philodendron?) vines will cascade. But it will still take some forethought and follow-through.

"Don't bite off more than you can chew," says Matt Kostelnick at Ambius. "Start with something smaller and see how that plant does. Remember—it's one thing to plant a garden; it's another thing to maintain it."

Even as a plant professional, Kostelnick says he, too, has been caught in the eyes-are-bigger-than-your-plate-of-succulents scenario when planning a summer vegetable garden. Start big and it just overwhelms you to the point where you can't properly care for any of your plants and probably forget about the whole thing while you're on vacation. He advises home gardeners to start small . . . and work their way up to the awesome jungles his company installs in buildings much bigger than your casa.

Kostelnick would guide plant newbies away from crotons and some palms because they tend to drop leaves at the first sign of stress. Or a weeping fig, which looks so pretty and outdoorsy when grown indoors but "will shed leaves when it gets cold, when it gets hot, when it gets dry, when you sneeze," he says. He's a big fan of pothos and philodendrons for first-timers: "They're easy to get, inexpensive, and last a long time; they're not fussy." Or you could try one of Kostelnick's favorite tropical alternatives to the vine plant, the dracaena.

DRACAENA

Or dracena, depending on whether you're the type of person who owns an encyclopaedia or encyclopedia. Although, does anyone actually use those anymore?

Dracaenas, or corn plants, make you feel like you're raising a palm, but they're a lot easier to deal with. They grow as high as four or six feet in indoor containers, rising from a central cane (what you'd call a trunk if you didn't know better) into long, narrow leaves reminiscent of those on a stalk of corn. They like a soothingly steady environment, so they're suited to the indoors. Just keep temperatures even, avoid direct sun, provide plenty of light, and use a pot that drains well.

Here's where they step out of the "easy starter" category: they can be a bit fussy with water. Unlike many of the plants we've profiled so far, they like a steadily moist soil. Not wet, moist. Moist, moist, moist. (Who here likes that word, besides dracaena?). You might also want to consider using distilled water, especially if your tap water is high in chlorine and fluoride. Dracaenas prefer a richer soil, so use a nutrient-dense potting soil to start and then fertilize during the summer growing season. If your dracaena is suffering from lack of humidity—perhaps in a really dry winter—set its pot in a tray of wet pebbles and lightly mist its long leaves.

The corn plant refers to *Dracaena fragrans*, a tropical African plant, but there are some other dracaena varieties that also add gorgeous foliage to your interior. Two of the more popular varieties are:

- *Dracaena marginata*: Also called the dragon tree, it's a little easier to deal with than a corn plant, gracefully tolerating temperature changes and drier soil. Its leaves grow in a spiky crown from a central stem; several stems grouped together can even be braided into a single thick and very cool-looking stem.
- *Dracaena deremensis*: This plant has the familiar corn-leaf style but grows in a stubbier, bushier shape than the popular stemmed varieties we've already covered. Distilled water and a humidity misting are also a good idea for this one.

Most of these easy-to-grow plants bring the peak of houseplant privileges. They look great, with that welcoming aloha vibe. They purify your indoor air, sucking in nasty toxins and pumping out gorgeous oxygen. They energize your mind and body with that unique verdant ability to connect you to the natural world.

Getting Started

If you have managed to bring up a sweet spider plant or a lovely little peace lily all on your own—with our guidance, of course—congratulations! We knew you could do it.

What happens, then, when you're ready to spread your rejuvenated plant spirit beyond the cast-iron plant pot? Is there a perfect plant for every nook and cranny?

Part 2

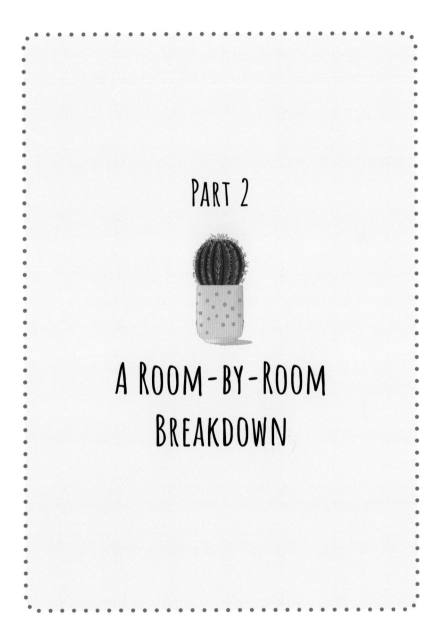

A Room-by-Room Breakdown

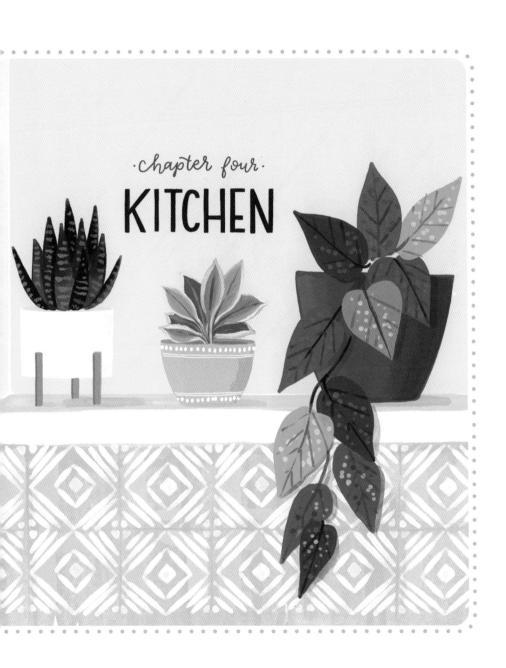

chapter four

KITCHEN

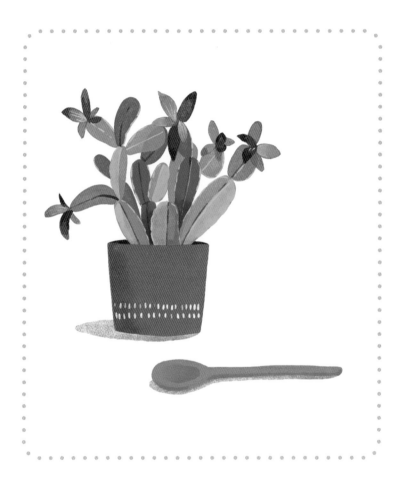

*F*irst stop on our tour: the kitchen.

For many of us—including a lot of current homebuilders and interior designers—the kitchen is the center of the home's activity. Whether it's your catchall for mail, bag, phone, keys, jacket . . . or where you laugh uproariously with fashionably dressed friends while sipping sauvignon blanc like those people in TV and magazine ads, this is going to be an important space for you: it's where you feed yourself.

What kitchens often have that other rooms may lack is a window and bright lights—even questionably skilled builders and architects seem to know cooking in the dark is a bit unwise. This direct source of light can give you opportunities for growing plants, whether for kitchen use or just kitchen kitsch that demands a lot of sunshine.

Your choice of houseplants for this space will no doubt reflect your choice for how to use this room. Are you an accomplished (or at least aspiring) gourmet cook? Your kitchen can be a great place to grow fresh herbs and other edibles to amplify your delicious creations! On the other hand, if your fanciest

> Bright lights are an edibles essential! If your kitchen is dim and your living room radiant, lead those tomato plants into the light.

cooking effort to date has been transferring kung pao takeout to a paper plate, your kitchen plants should veer toward the stylish rather than the functional.

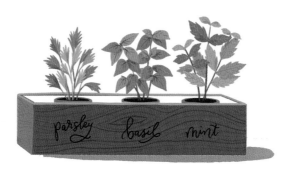

HERBAL REMEDIES

Harvesting is an extremely satisfying experience. When your daily life looks like an in-box that is always full, you have an unending list of chores, and every meeting you attend wraps up with "let's circle back to this," it can be deeply satisfying to pluck a sprig of mint from your own plant and say: *I made this.* In a doubtful world, this is a real thing.

Herbs make the ideal start to a kitchen garden because they are relatively easy to grow. They need lots of bright sunshine, and because that makes for warm work, they need regular watering. If you can supply those necessities, you can be an herb farmer. Got a bright kitchen windowsill? A countertop or wall flooded with light? That's everything *and* the kitchen sink (which, since it is bound to be close by, makes the perfect place to water and drain your herb garden).

There are two sources for starting an indoor herb garden: from plants or from seeds. Which you choose depends in part on what kind of herbs you want to grow. Popular herbs like basil are widely available in plant form and grow quickly when transplanted at home. Starting from seeds will, of course, take longer to get a productive plant, but it gives you the opportunity to try unique and hard-to-find herbs: sweet basil, Thai basil, opal basil, lemon basil, holy basil, spicy globe basil—you could become a total basil snob and irritate/impress your friends with exotic basil options.

> Herb gardens don't require a ton of room! If your kitchen counter space is at a premium, a windowsill garden or even small pots hanging from hooks near your window will do the job.

If you start with young plants, they can be planted and cared for like most houseplants: good potting mix and a well-draining pot will take you far. Wait until the plant is well established in its new home and producing new growth before you start cooking with it.

If you start with seeds, get your pot ready to go by filling it with damp potting mix up to an inch below the rim. Sprinkle in a few seeds (not the whole packet!) and then cover them with a little extra potting mix. Covering the container with plastic wrap can help lock in moisture while they germinate. Until these seeds have sprouted and rooted, be very careful with watering so they aren't displaced. They are babies. Be gentle.

Whether starting from plant or seed, which herbs should you grow? Because this is a useful houseplant, not just a decorative one, pick herbs that you actually enjoy. If cilantro tastes like soap to you, don't grow cilantro.

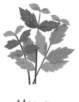

MINT

Bloomscape's Joyce Mast puts mint at the top of the indoor kitchen garden list. "Mint is a fun, easy-to-grow herb. It grows quickly and smells great. There are many uses for mint, including adding it to drinks, tea, or dishes."

It's best to keep mint in its own container, not mixed with other herbs, because it is not a good sharer. It will eagerly and rapidly gobble up an entire pot, even sending off overflow shoots into neighboring pots. If plants ever take over the earth, they will probably be led by mint.

Mint is best started from a plant, not a seed. It doesn't require as much sun as most herbs, so a windowsill or space with indirect light will work just fine. Water when the top inch of soil is dry and make sure it drains completely. Mist the mint if your climate is especially dry. When harvesting your mint, be prepared to be ruthless! Generous cutting keeps its growth in check. If this necessitates a generous julep to celebrate harvest day, so be it.

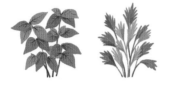

Basil and Parsley

These are great plants to start from either seedling or seed and grow well together if you decide on a pot-sharing arrangement. Both will want a minimum of six hours of bright sun, and they like to stay hydrated, so keep the soil moist but drained. They will rot from the roots in wet soil, but they won't take in soil nutrients if the soil is dry.

Harvest vigorously! These plants grow fuller and bushier if you regularly snip sprigs. Be aware, though, that these are annuals, not perennials, meaning that unlike some plants that will grow happily year after year, you should expect these to last a season before you discard them. Eventually—and more quickly if you don't prune—they flower and the flavor of their leaves diminishes. When that happens, it's time to start over with new plants—and that's totally okay. You haven't failed; you have successfully guided them through their life cycle.

Other good options in the annual or seasonal herb category include: chives, nasturtiums, cilantro, dill.

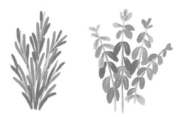

Rosemary and Oregano

These are called "woody herbs" for their stems, which are more like sticks than tender shoots. It's best to start these from a seedling or cutting, not seeds. They can last a long time, even years, if well tended. Like the previously listed herbs, they will require a ton of sun, but keep them on the drier side in a sand-based potting soil that drains efficiently. Because they will be keeping you company for a long time, you will want to think about repotting annually. If you're using them regularly in your elegant cuisine, they'll be trimmed well and grow into beautiful, shapely plants that lend a light perfume to your kitchen.

> These are only a few options. Seed shop online and you'll find dozens of unusual and hard-to-find herb varieties.

Veg Out

Having mastered the herb garden, are you ready for your next crop? How about tomatoes and peppers? Both on the easier side of indoor gardening, these plants pair nicely with all those beautiful herbs you've been producing.

What you will need is sunshine, making this a more successful undertaking in summer months, when there's just more sunshine around. You'll need to give them as much as ten hours of bright sun a day to get fruit (yes, both tomatoes and peppers are fruit) growing, whether you're starting from seedlings or seeds. Containers should be at least twelve inches deep; you won't want to try repotting them when they're full of fruit. Keep soil at a consistent dampness, and fertilize once a week with a product designed for vegetables. Also, be ready with stakes or tomato cages because they will grow fast and need lots of physical, not just emotional, support when they're top-heavy with fruit.

A few awkward words about reproduction. You know about the birds and the bees, right? Well, for the indoor fruiting plant, that's you. This is a relatively unembarrassing situation with peppers—they are self-pollinating, and just ruffling their blooms will make those little peppers grow. You will need to be more diligent about "manual pollination" with the demure tomato plant. If the jostle isn't working, try nudging pollen onto the stamen with a cotton swab or toothpick. Always ask permission first.

If you're looking for the fastest-growing indoor veg, starting microgreens or lettuce from seed will get you a quick, if limited, crop.

You can get as ambitious as your patience and space allow for your indoor victory garden project, but remember that elaborate home farming does tend to require more elaborate equipment. Vegetables can be demanding roommates: they take up a lot of space. While peppers and some tomatoes are relatively compact, zucchini and squash grow wide bushes, and cucumbers or other vines need to be confined to trellises.

Grow lights, hydroponic towers, indoor grow kits—these and every other trick you find shopping online can work for an indoor farm garden, but it's definitely a setup for the committed gardener. Mary Beth Shaddix of Maple Valley Nursery discourages newbie plant parents from going all in on these fancy setups right away: "I would ding it for impracticality. It can turn into a pricey project."

The bottom line? Grow what makes sense for your time, budget, and taste buds. A few well-placed pots can go a long way to improving your meals year-round. And you don't need to check the *Farmers' Almanac* to know that.

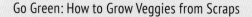

Go Green: How to Grow Veggies from Scraps

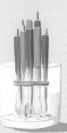

Is there anything more environmentally hip than recycling even your plants? If you're looking for a little entertainment in the kitchen or want to save a little money by stretching your produce, join the trend of people growing new plants from kitchen scraps.

Now, this won't work effectively with every vegetable—for example, don't bury a piece of broccoli and expect a full new head to grow. There are, however, a few popular choices that do well at growing new roots from scraps, including scallions (green onions), celery, carrots, pineapple, potatoes, and herbs.

The procedure is straightforward, if a little time-consuming. New plants can grow from roots, from a cutting, or from an "eye," so to get started, you'll want to create the right kind of scraps:

- **Scallions**: Cut off about one inch of the white part of the scallion, including the roots. Set the rooted end in enough water to cover the roots, but not the whole scrap. New green growth will emerge from the cut end. This also works with a leek or the top of a whole bulb onion.

- **Pineapple**: Cut the top, including the leaves, off a whole pineapple, including about one-half inch of fruit.
- **Celery and bok choy**: Cut off the stalks, leaving about two inches of the base.
- **Carrots and beets**: Cut the top off a whole carrot or beet (this won't work with "baby carrots" from a bag).
- **Herbs**: If you're using a grocery store bunch, use a leftover sprig.
- **Potatoes and sweet potatoes**: If you've ever forgotten about a potato in the back of a cupboard, you probably have already seen it grow nubs or sprouts from its eyes. Cut a chunk of potato that includes that eye.

Once you have your scrap, set it in a container and add just enough water to cover the cut end. You should *not* cover the whole scrap (and if you're growing an herb, you should be sure to keep any leaves out of the water as well). Change the water daily to prevent bacteria growth, and watch small white roots begin to emerge from your new plant!

When the roots or stalks growing from this recycled rubbish are an inch long, you can pot them in potting soil and grow them as you would any other plant. Some of them will grow into new and useful replicas of themselves (carrots and celery), while others (like onions) will grow flower stalks and give you some free seeds from whence you'll have a whole new garden. Prepare the salad bowl!

But let's be clear about this: the point is not that you will never have to buy produce again. Your crop will be limited, but there can be something deeply satisfying about stretching your produce a bit further and getting the most from every scallion. Waste not, want not and all that. If you get joy in propagating new plants from old, go for it! But if you envision yourself as a farmer, maybe stick to the more realistic herb garden.

No, Not Dessert—We Said "Desert"

So maybe you're not much of a cook. A home-cooked meal at your place is microwaving last night's leftover pizza. Why would you want to grow herbs or vegetables when you'll never use them? But you don't let your "opinionated" older sister belittle your cooking skill-lessness, so instead you use your disinterest in sautéing and stewing to inspire your own kitchen style.

Introducing the cactus, Mother Earth's reminder to get out of the way and mind your own business.

Cacti demand the same kind of bright sunshine that benefits the aforementioned edible gardens, but they do a much better job clarifying to guests that your kitchen was meant for a chic, clean look, not an up-to-your-elbows-in-dirty-pots-and-pans look.

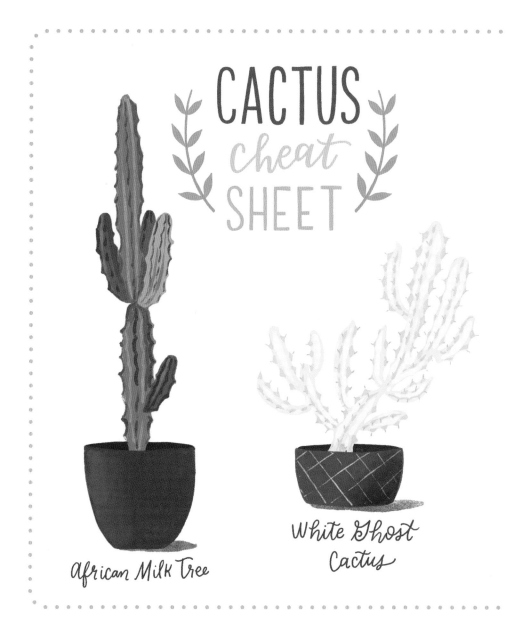

CACTUS
cheat
SHEET

African Milk Tree

White Ghost
Cactus

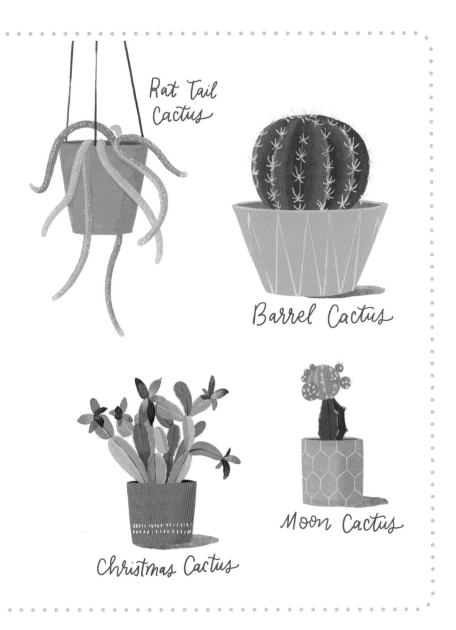

Rat Tail Cactus

Barrel Cactus

Christmas Cactus

Moon Cactus

According to Crystal Desi, owner of succulent and cactus plant store Cactus Moon in Florida, a lot of cacti do well as indoor plants. Much like succulents (all cacti are succulents; not all succulents are cacti—it's a square-rectangle kinda thing), they don't require extensive watering or lots of dusting and pruning. "Place it in a corner and just let it alone!" says Desi.

Find your cactus a spot with that popular bright, indirect light. Desi suggests a kitchen window or even an interior space that is consistently well lit. "As long as your plants are getting six hours of light—even incandescent light—they're fine," she says.

Potting soil should be selected carefully for cacti. Regular potting soil tends to retain moisture to keep tropical plant roots damp, but a cactus will rot in wet soil. Use a special cactus potting soil that drains quickly, and make sure your pot will let water flow through. You will only want to water a cactus when the soil around it is completely dry, "when it feels like sand," says Desi.

Desi's favorite indoor cacti include the white ghost cactus (a pale gray-green candelabra shape with pink flowers) and the African milk tree (also called a cathedral cactus, with small green leaves growing among thorns on tall, straight arms). If you're looking for a variety that takes up less floor space—more of a countertop companion—try one of these smaller cacti:

Barrel cactus, or golden barrel cactus, is an adorable little ball of brutally sharp needles. Its center is a juicy green, but you'll never get that

> **Cactus Cheat Sheet:**
>
> • Provide bright light.
> • Water when soil is very dry.
> • Pot in cactus soil to help it dry out between waterings.

close—clusters of long spines sprout from evenly spaced knobs from every curve. It's pleasingly symmetrical in appearance and perfectly round when it's young. It's nicknamed "mother-in-law's cushion." A useful plant.

Moon cactus is a strange one to care for because it is actually two plants in one. The top (properly named *Gymnocalycium*, but that's a mouthful for something as cutely named as "moon cactus") gives the species its other name, ruby ball cactus . . . though sometimes that top is in fact yellow. Whether vivid red or vivid yellow, it appears as a ball shape, popping out smaller balls with little spines. The bright top is albino and produces no plant food—chlorophyll—of its own, so it is grafted to a second, more productive plant. This is usually a thick green column with a few small spines. Being different creatures, the two halves of the cactus have somewhat different needs. Defer to the base rootstock; it's the hardworking, food-producing half of the partnership, while the ball just sits around looking pretty. Give the rootstock lots of light. Water only when totally dry, waiting until it's even a little wilted just to be extra sure. If it drains well, your cactus will plump back up.

Rat tail cactus earns its unfortunate name, producing long trailing stems covered with tiny bristles. It looks like something you may not want to encounter unexpectedly in an eighties hairstyle, but as a houseplant, it makes a distinctive statement. Great on a counter, a windowsill, or as a hanging plant (those "tails" can grow to four feet!), it will need plenty of direct sunshine and can handle a little forgetfulness on watering. It also likes to be repotted regularly because producing a rat tail apparently takes a lot of nutrients. Give it new soil annually, even if it's not yet ready for a bigger pot. Expect fabulous hot-pink flowers, something that can't be said of more literal rat tails.

All of the above are desert cacti, but there are also cacti of tropical origins if you want a less bristly cactus for a close-quartered kitchen.

Christmas cactus grows in wide, flat, toothed stem segments that, when it blooms, end in scarlet flowers. In the Northern Hemisphere, it flowers in the winter, hence its seasonal name. In its native Brazil, it's called the *flor de Maio*, the May flower. This plant has, of course, very different needs from its desert cousins. Water it well when its stems look limp, but make sure it drains thoroughly. Give it less light and more humidity; it will be happy on a kitchen counter and getting an occasional misting. Cut its daily light supply starting in October (provide twelve to fourteen hours of darkness) and it may reward you with some midwinter holiday blooms.

Cacti are statement plants for sure. It takes confidence and a certain prickliness of character to make them the focus of your kitchen decor. If you like the fierce look but are in search of a kinder, gentler friend, **aloe** may be a more nurturing place to start. After all, the aloe vera variety will quite literally care for your body, while its more colorful cousins can add decorative intrigue.

Better still, aloe is *extremely* easy to care for. Desi would even go so far as to say you can neglect it.

You've probably already seen the aloe vera, a memorable succulent whose leaf gel saved you that time you forgot to wear sunscreen at the beach (ouch). Aloe vera produces long, thick, spined leaves from its soil-level base. To thrive, it needs bright light but not direct sunshine, advice you probably should follow yourself if you don't want to use too many of its leaves for medicinal purposes. Water when the soil is dried out and drain it thoroughly. Pot it in cactus or succulent soil to help it drain efficiently and pick a wide rather than deep pot; aloe's roots grow along the surface.

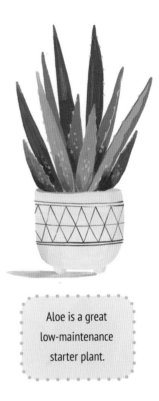

Harvesting the gel is simple. First, wait until you burn yourself. Second, cut a leaf from the plant near where it meets the stem and squeeze out the interior gel to rub over your burn. The plant will grow new leaves and you will grow new skin. For such a sharp-looking plant, it's a real

Aloe is a great low-maintenance starter plant.

sweetie pie. Keep in mind that aloe vera gel is *soothing*, but there's not a lot of research showing that it's *healing*. Don't confuse it with a real doctor.

Of course, aloe vera is not the only aloe. There are hundreds of varieties with fewer followers that may not produce soothing gel but do have a similarly sculptural aesthetic. They all tend to feature the tooth-edged succulent leaves that rise in a rosette pattern from the base, but those leaves can be pink or purple, silver or green, spiraling in patterns, or growing spiky flowers. An option for every style!

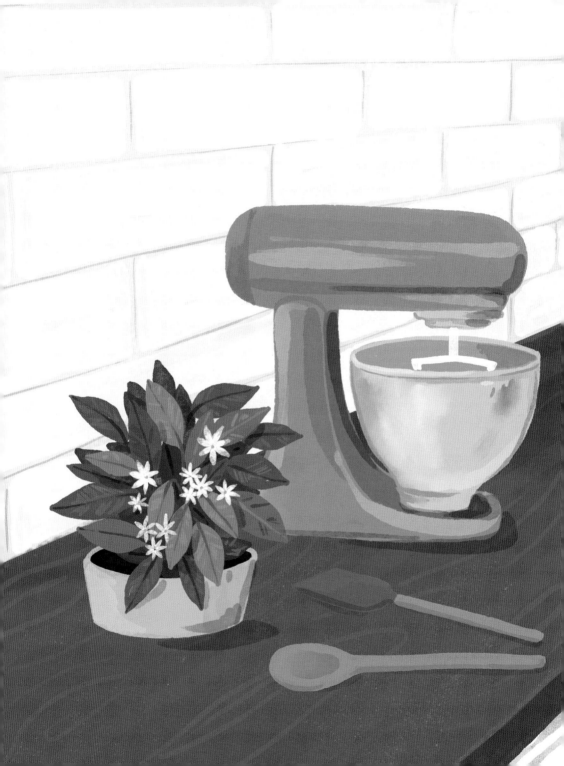

Make Your Kitchen a No-Stress Zone

Herbs, vegetables, cactus, aloe—your kitchen has turned into a busy place. But that's not the same thing as a stressful place. Getting a meal on the table can be a project, even if it's just for yourself, and even if you're an accomplished chef. Coming home to unwashed dishes at the end of a workday wears everyone out. Calling your favorite takeout place only to discover the health department shut them down last week is disheartening. The kitchen is a work space and its insistence on utilitarian activities can overwhelm even the most Zen among us.

This is where your houseplants come in. Gardening—indoors or out—reduces stress.

Stress is tremendously debilitating to your health, both physical and mental, but our efficient modern lifestyles frequently demand stressful activity—jobs, relationships, commutes—all at a hectic pace.

Unlike a plant, we can't just shed a yellow leaf to call out for help when we're stressed. We make ourselves ill, we lash out at those who love us, we fall short of our best selves. Time to hug a houseplant! Studies published in the *Journal of Health Psychology* show that gardening reduces cortisol (that's the stress hormone) levels, and that people report feeling more positive and happier after spending as little as thirty minutes gardening. As you water your herb garden or check your cactus for good drainage, you are similarly feeding and tending to your own health. Even just looking at a beautiful living bit of greenery will soothe the savage beast within.

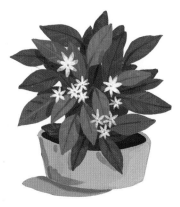

Jasmine

Jasmine is perfect for some indoor gardening beauty because it's a plant that's as sweetly fragrant as it is good-lookin'. Climbing, twining, and trailing long vines with glossy dark-green leaves and scattered with tiny star-shaped white blossoms, jasmine can frame your kitchen space with a rewarding beauty. It's not designed for utilitarian use like aloe vera or an edible garden. Please don't eat it. This one is to feed your spirit.

Jasmine looks to the light. Lots and lots of light. This plant is a natural sunbather, but it prefers damp soil at all times. Now, that's *damp*, not soaked, so give it good drainage. When lots of new leaves and new vines show up during the growing season, prune it to make sure it focuses its strength on its climbing vines, not on creating new shoots. It blooms in the winter months; support its flowering with a nitrogen-light fertilizer and a snug pot. If you're having trouble getting it to bloom, trick it into thinking winter has begun by cutting back on its light sources: close some blinds, or put it in a shady corner for a few days.

There are several varieties of jasmine that do well indoors, but they all grow differently so pick one that fits what you're looking for. Climbing varieties like *Jasminum* or Chinese or star jasmine have an appealing look, but if your space and style are not suited to vines, there are shrub jasmine plants as well, such as orange jasmine.

Jasmine flowers produce a heady, almost indecent perfume that is particularly sweet at night, perfect for giving your midnight snacks a scent of mystery and romance. Breathe deep, de-stress, and help yourself to the ice cream.

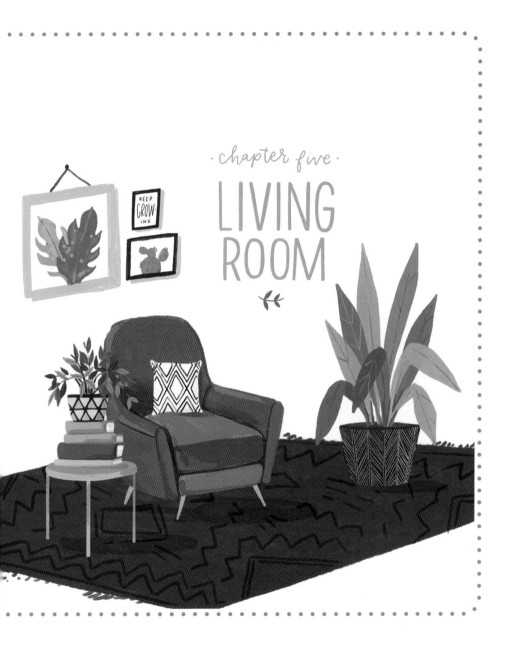

chapter five

LIVING
ROOM

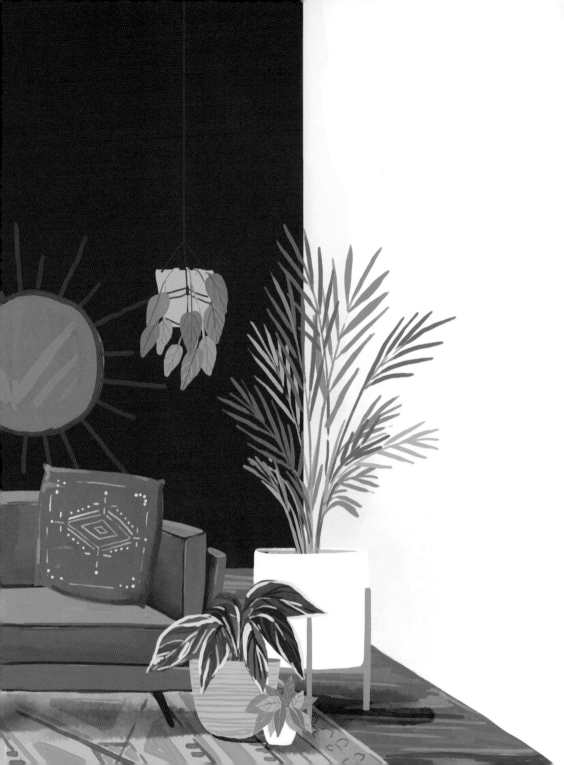

The living room can be a rather undefined space in your home if you let it. You cook in the kitchen, you sleep in the bedroom, you work in the office, you bathe in the bathroom. Sure, let's "live" in the living room, but apart from plunking down a couch and a TV, how you fill the empty space will determine what that living looks like.

Whether you have a twenty-room mansion or your tiny apartment could fit in that mansion's coat closet, your living room is the space where you spend most of your nonsleeping time. Decorating the space to make it welcoming to friends, family, and especially yourself is not a side hobby; it's a moment of self-definition. You'll want to choose furniture, knick-knacks, and, yes, houseplants that will reflect your idea of comfort and energy.

Your living room is where your public and private lives meet. This is where you can welcome friends, entertain, wine, and dine. This is also where you can step away from outside life and hibernate with a good book and a cup of tea. It would be really weird to try to enjoy both aspects of your life in your bathroom, for example, but the living room is designed for your full range of living.

That makes it a natural place to include plants—nothing like something alive to help your room feel truly lived in.

"When choosing a plant, pick one that speaks to your home's personality, but also consider how it will thrive in the environment you provide," says Joyce Mast. The goal is to balance the aesthetic you want with the practical limitations of your room.

So what *is* your home's personality? What kind of environment can you provide? Let's get set up for A+ plant parenthood:

- What do you want your living space to say about you? Decide early on whether you want your space to scream "urban jungle" or just prove to your mom that you can keep something alive.
- How do you use this space? TV time? Reading nooks? Clutter magnet strewn with the kids' toys? Entertaining friends?
- Where might a plant fit? Corners? Bookshelves and mantels? Picture window? Side tables?
- What kind of light do you have? Lots of bright sunshine or dim and mysterious?
- What's the air circulation like? An AC vent blasting into a room can be overwhelmingly breezy for tropical plants, but if your space gets a little musty from lack of airflow, plants that rely on good air movement (like air plants!) will struggle.
- Is the room humid or more arid? And not just the room—what is your region's climate like? It can be hard to supply enough damp air for a fern in a

desert, but in humid climates, you'll have to keep an eye out for fungus growth on your plants.

If these seem like a lot of questions to keep track of just to get a houseplant, that's because creating balance is both the goal and the purpose of your main living area at home.

And not to get too fêng shui on you, but including houseplants in your living room design creates an additional element of balance, bringing that all-important "wood element" inside. Nature feeds the human spirit. "To the body and mind which have been cramped by noxious work or company, nature is medicinal and restores their tone," as Ralph Waldo Emerson wrote. Though the four walls of habitation block out that nature, even the most modest of African violets can bridge the gap and offer you outside solace for inside life.

Larger houseplants can also add a sculptural element to those empty spaces. Too large a room to be cozy? Use a big houseplant to demarcate living zones, separate entryway from living room from dining room. Too tiny a space to fit more than that couch? A taller houseplant draws the eyes upward, making better use of vertical space and giving the area a more open feel.

WELCOME HOME, WANDERER

When you return home, exhausted from your travels and travails, what better botanic friend could you have to greet you than Ulysses?

Ulysses, also known as *Dracaena warneckii*, is not unfamiliar—we mentioned other dracaena varieties in chapter 3—but in this particular guise, it's especially well-suited to beginning your houseplant decorating career. You can put it in a corner, set it in an entryway, or tuck it behind the couch and it will be just fine without excessive attention.

"It's highly adaptable and easy to care for," says Plant Mom Joyce Mast. "They thrive on neglect, adapt to low-light conditions, and they do not like to be overwatered."

Of course, it will capture your attention anyway because it's a fantastic plant. The statuesque, narrow shape lends itself to a corner and smaller living spaces. Its habit of stripping the air around it of toxins like benzene, formaldehyde, xylene, and toluene likewise lends itself to indoor popularity.

A relative of the corn plant, this is a tall, bushy plant with long, draping leaves striped in shiny dark green and white sprouting from canes. Water when the top inch of soil is dry, and *only* when the top inch is dry. Good drainage is important! Ulysses can grow to over four feet tall, so repotting can be challenging but necessary when it outgrows its pot.

Plants like Ulysses make a statement. And that's just what a living room needs: a statement that sets the tone of the room. If Ulysses isn't the statement you had in mind, though, there are plenty of other striking houseplants from which to choose when you're ready to voyage on.

Buy a **parlor palm** and, just like that, your humdrum living room is a parlor. Should you serve tea? Is the vicar

> Drainage reminder! Don't let water collect in the bottom of a pot. Let it flow....

calling? These are questions you'll have to answer yourself, but we can tell you that the lush green fronds on groupings of slender stems have been popular as indoor plants since they graced nineteenth-century parlors (hence the name).

Mast describes the parlor palm as a graceful and easy compact palm that thrives in a variety of light situations and tight spaces. More light will encourage it to grow faster, but it will adapt to low light. It would rather be too dry than too wet, so don't water until its top layer of soil is completely dry. It won't need to be repotted often, if ever, so consider whatever stylish pot you select for it as a stable part of your home decor.

Bamboo palms, which have a similar look but are more robust in stature than the parlor palm, are a good alternative. "This plant will bring color and warmth to your room. It's a statement piece for the corner," Mast says. **Areca palms** will need more light than either the parlor palm or bamboo palm but fill a sunny corner with a comparable tropical grandeur.

Ficus has a long and checkered history as a houseplant. On the plus side, it is the tree under which Buddha sat when he achieved enlightenment. On the negative side, it's picky and demanding. But then, so is enlightenment. If you can't remember to water your ficus, are you likely to be one who remembers to nurture your inner Buddha?

Ficus Cheat Sheet

- Medium light
- Regular watering
- Frequent fertilizing
- Dependable care

The **rubber plant**, *Ficus elastica*, is a gorgeous starting point, with big, shiny green leaves offset by reddish stems and leaf veins. It can grow up to fifty feet in its natural tropical environment but will agree to a smaller stature when you can only offer nine-foot ceilings. Like most ficus plants, it likes to keep moist, so consistent watering is a must. It also likes consistent fertilizing, preferring a weak solution. Give it consistent sunshine, not too bright or direct. "Consistency" is the watchword here. If you can be reliable and attentive, your rubber plant will adapt to the indoor life. If you can't stick to a pattern, a sickly rubber plant won't easily bounce back.

Balance is similarly necessary for the *Ficus benjamina*, the **weeping fig**. With smaller, daintier leaves than the rubber plant, it grows branches, giving you the look of a deciduous shade tree indoors. It is a bit of a Goldilocks, though, and will lose its leaves if it is too wet or too dry, too bright or too dark. It doesn't like to be moved, either, so find it a spot where it can stay indefinitely. No need to weep; this fig is a beautiful, reliable friend as long as you are, too.

Time to talk about the elephant in the room: the **fiddle-leaf fig tree**. Of course you love it. Just like you love boy bands. Being too popular and overplayed isn't the *Ficus lyrata*'s fault any more than it is Harry Styles's. If you just have to have a fiddle-leaf fig tree, go for it and ignore the haters saying, "Oh, another one?" But know what you're in for. Like a boy band star, this fig is fickle. It wanted to retire to a garden in Florida, but since you have installed it in your living room, be prepared to pamper. Provide steady moisture, bright light (but not too intense—east-facing windows are usually a hit), reliable warmth, and frequent misting for humidity, and dust those leaves. But even the biggest fangirl/boy can fall short for this one. When a leaf is injured, bruised, or bitten by a pest, ugly brown spots appear. It can also get fungal diseases, aphids, mealy bugs, and the like.

If you can make this work, the results will be awesome. Fiddle-leaf fig trees grow quickly to a full six feet. You can repot it while it's young and still small enough to manipulate—and those roots grow *fast*, so it's necessary. When it gets too statuesque for repotting, gently scrape out old soil from around the roots and add some fresh stuff for an annual nutrient boost that will keep it gorgeous and popular for years to come.

Some people opt for columns and chandeliers; you went with palms and ficus to add statement decor of dimension and opulence. Now let's add "the look."

Look at Me, Look at Me!

When you feel ready for a look somewhat more sophisticated than a collection of Precious Moments figurines, turn to the kind of houseplants that can add a design element to your living room with flair and drama. These are the houseplants you can't take your eyes off: the vividly colored, the statuesque, the purely entertaining.

To start with a little color, start with a **croton**. There are hundreds of varieties of this tropical plant from Southeast Asia, and you have probably seen them as popular indoor planter fillers in malls and public buildings. Their thick, shiny leaves lend a polished, finished appearance to your room, but the best part of crotons is that they come in a dazzling array of colors to match whatever decorative theme you've got going: green, of course, but also orange, red, and yellow. It's the brilliance of fall foliage all year long, right in your own home!

Croton gets its name from the Greek word for tick, referring to the appearance of its seed. But croton can be a real tick. This qualifies as a higher-maintenance plant. Like the ficus varieties, crotons like regular watering so the soil stays moist but not wet enough to cause root rot. If you have a particularly dry environment (you live in a dry climate or your heating system dries out the winter air indoors), misting is a good idea. If it gets too dry, the croton is susceptible to spider mites. If being picky about moisture isn't enough, the croton also has some specific lighting demands: lots of it. Select a spot near a window and add regular dusting to your routine, since the croton's leathery leaves do need to be wiped down to be able to take in enough sunlight. Not enough sun? Say goodbye to those bright colors—they will fade without enough light.

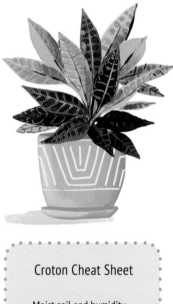

Croton Cheat Sheet

- Moist soil and humidity
- Bright light
- Regular dusting

Once these needs are met, however, a croton will add an unforgettable burst of color to your room. They usually grow to about three feet high indoors and are full and leafy. Have some fun with this one—crotons' leaf shapes are as uniquely varied as their hues: oval, narrow, or twisted. Select from its great varietal names like Dreadlocks, Mona Lisa, Petra, and so many more.

If, however, all these demanding ficus plants and crotons are wearing you out—all you really wanted to do in your living room was relax after a long day—order up a **peperomia** and chill.

No, peperomia is not a pizza topping. It's an epiphytic South American rain forest transplant that's having a bit of a moment as a houseplant, probably because it offers the colorful variety of a croton without the neediness.

The thousands of varieties of peperomia feature thick, fleshy leaves with interesting textures and dramatic colors like red, green, silver, or purple. Some leaves are big, some are small; you pick which is just right for you. The varieties of peperomia include:

- Belly button: small clusters of tiny leaves
- Suzanne: deeply ridged leaves brushed with silver
- Cupid: heart-shaped, cream-edged leaves on trailing stems

Whatever style you select, your peperomia comes with a very simple care list. Like an orchid, it is accustomed to growing on tree branches or other small perches, not in soil; plant it in an orchid potting mix in a fast-draining pot. Only water it when the soil is completely dry, which means that if you forget occasionally, it will be just fine! It needs that bright, indirect (medium) lighting typical of rain forest dwellers and only rarely will want fertilizing. It prefers to be rootbound. Repot when roots start growing out of drainage holes, but otherwise let it snuggle in. Sometimes called "baby rubber plant" (though it is not, in fact, at all related to the rubber plant), peperomia is more of a tabletop or shelf plant in size, giving it its other nickname, radiator plant.

Size Doesn't Matter

Tucked into corners, appearing unexpectedly among coffee-table books and picture frames, delicate small plants lend your room a personal feeling because they are so clearly chosen for individual taste, not as space fillers or even for their health benefits.

Here are a few display options to help petite plants make a big statement:

1. **The gang's all here.** When grouped, houseplants can provide a green backdrop to brighten your home decor and lift your home's energy. You display all those family photos in a row on your mantelpiece; time to display the family houseplants with as much thoughtfulness and affection. There are two main things to keep in mind when grouping several houseplants: the look and the location.

Make sure your plants look good together—no one wants to be the one in the relationship that makes everyone think, "How did *he* get *her?*" Taller plants should stand in the back row, just like in class photos, so their shadows don't diminish smaller plants' photosynthesis ability. Put those more colorful plants to the front so their brilliance is undiminished. Add a variety of textures and heights to keep it interesting.

But as good as plants look with each other, they should also share some complementary habits. Plants that like humidity love being in a group (they can enjoy one another's respiration). Plants that like the same amount of sunlight are going to like sharing the same spot on the windowsill. Plants from a shared background (tropical rain forest, desert plains) tend to match well.

2. **Contain your excitement.** For an even chummier group, why not let several plants share the same pot? This is not the same as having to share a bedroom with your sister when you were a kid. The right selection of plants can share one pot without fighting. But be strategic; potting a ficus with a cactus is just not going to work—one loves water, one avoids it. Pick plants that need the same amount of sunshine, are on the same watering cycle, and use the same soil type.

After you've grouped responsibly, you can have a little fun. Play with heights; play with textures; play with colors. Here are a few ideas, but possibilities are endless:

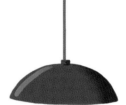

- Parlor palm, maidenhair fern, creeping fig
- Moth orchids, pothos, Spanish moss
- Snake plant, pencil cactus, echeveria, string of pearls
- Bromeliad vriesea, cupid peperomia, lemon-lime philodendron

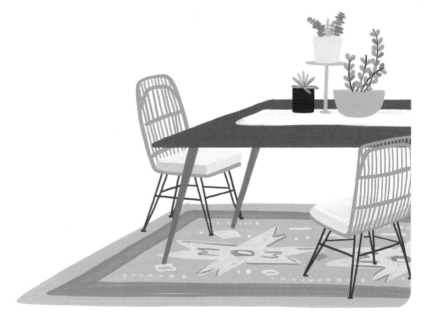

3. **The glass is half full.** When you've mastered the container garden, it's time to graduate to the sophisticated but super simple terrarium. Its glass enclosure gives this plant home an elegance that makes it ideal for a dining room table centerpiece. And that protective glass shell gives you a little more freedom in plant options if you're trying to keep toxic plants away from pets or small children.

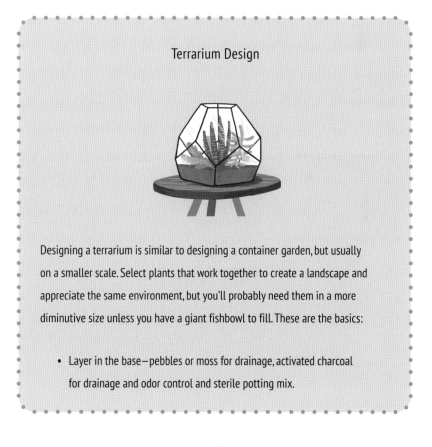

Terrarium Design

Designing a terrarium is similar to designing a container garden, but usually on a smaller scale. Select plants that work together to create a landscape and appreciate the same environment, but you'll probably need them in a more diminutive size unless you have a giant fishbowl to fill. These are the basics:

- Layer in the base—pebbles or moss for drainage, activated charcoal for drainage and odor control and sterile potting mix.

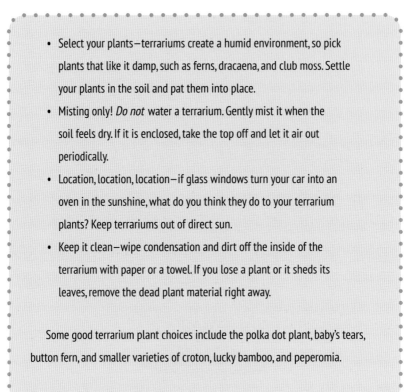

- Select your plants—terrariums create a humid environment, so pick plants that like it damp, such as ferns, dracaena, and club moss. Settle your plants in the soil and pat them into place.
- Misting only! *Do not* water a terrarium. Gently mist it when the soil feels dry. If it is enclosed, take the top off and let it air out periodically.
- Location, location, location—if glass windows turn your car into an oven in the sunshine, what do you think they do to your terrarium plants? Keep terrariums out of direct sun.
- Keep it clean—wipe condensation and dirt off the inside of the terrarium with paper or a towel. If you lose a plant or it sheds its leaves, remove the dead plant material right away.

Some good terrarium plant choices include the polka dot plant, baby's tears, button fern, and smaller varieties of croton, lucky bamboo, and peperomia.

Fancy Plants

You've added grand statement plants, you've added stirring colors, you've added the delicate small touches. Let's keep it fun and add a little whimsy.

Staghorn fern is an air plant, so this is a fun one for playing around with the display. Hanging baskets will work, but heavy pots of soil will not. Try a wall mount instead! Pick your base, whether it's a board or a piece of driftwood, and nail a small circle of flat-headed nails around the area where you want to attach your fern. In the center, mound some potting mix and wet sphagnum moss to make a bed for your fern. Set the fern on its bed and layer additional moss over the roots. Weave fishing twine or wire between the nails, across the moss and fern roots, to secure it into place. To water a mounted fern, you'll need to get the whole moss apparatus thoroughly wet about once a week and mist it periodically. Now you have the long, jagged fronds of a fern to hang from your wall. Some people hang deer antlers over the mantelpiece. You hang staghorn ferns. No animals were harmed in the making of this decor.

Swiss cheese plant, or *Monstera adansonii*, has large heart-shaped leaves speckled with the holes that give it its name. This is a good climbing plant, and the more it climbs, the larger its leaves; the larger its leaves, the more holes appear. Give it a climbing trellis, indirect light, and consistently moist soil. It may even be your best conversation piece: "My mom asked me before in all seriousness if I had cut the holes in my *Monstera adansonii* leaves," says Joyce Mast.

Ponytail palm, a vigorous sprout of fine, curling palm fronds atop a bulbous trunk, brings the fun without bringing the work. "It is ideal for people who have little time or travel frequently," says Mast. "It requires very little care, as it is drought tolerant and slow-growing. It only needs watering every couple of weeks (its bulblike trunk stores water), sparingly in the winter months, and can be left alone to soak up the sunlight." All the perky cuteness of a high ponytail or a pom-pom without the cheerleader. Go team palm!

Tying It Together

In every successful gathering space, there is that ineffable something that brings the disparate parts into a unified theme. Of course, your naturally sparkling personality will set the ambience, but don't turn down a little help from your houseplant. What better plant to tie it all together than the climbing plant, literally twining and binding furniture and foliage in a cohesive greenery.

Passionflower: This vine runs rampant, a glory of green leaves and delicate, twisting stems—if you're lucky, it will flower, too. Its flowers are usually white and purple, arranged in a series of petals and sepals that are said to symbolize the Passion of Christ (hence its name). Whatever its religious significance, be ready with a climbing apparatus (a trellis? a curtain rod? a piece of furniture that can get viney?), because it grows fast and furious. Outdoors, it can grow so rapidly that some regions have labeled it an invasive species, but you can keep an eye on the invader successfully inside. Be ruthless in your pruning. Show that vine who's boss.

Passionflower vines of different varieties produce different colors of blooms: purple, white, blue, or red. Some types even grow an edible fruit! Lots of sunlight, lots of water, rich soil, and regular fertilizing will encourage it to bloom in the summer months.

Whatever plant (or plants!) you choose, your spirit can be revived by the newfound peace of your own living room. Successfully deploying house-plants in your decorating scheme gives your home that positive energy of light filtered through greenery, old furniture brightened by a leafy companion, tabletops warmed with color and texture. Your plants help you steady your course between the pressures of life and the pressures of home to create a balanced, rewarding space for yourself, family, and friends.

When you are retreating to your personal oasis, shutting out the problems of the outside world, your houseplants let the natural world in for some organic rejuvenation in the midst of your sanctuary.

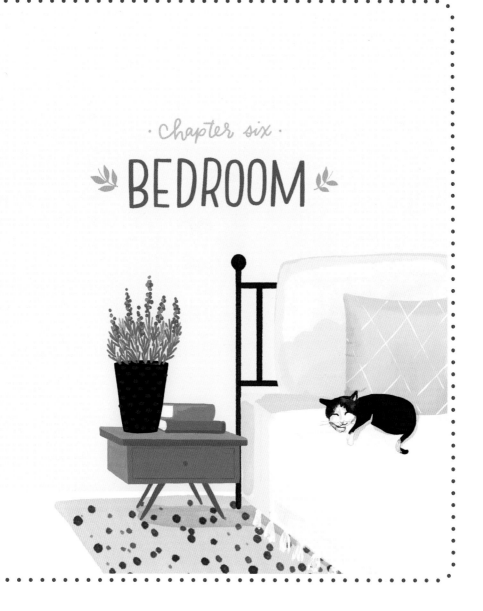

· chapter six ·

BEDROOM

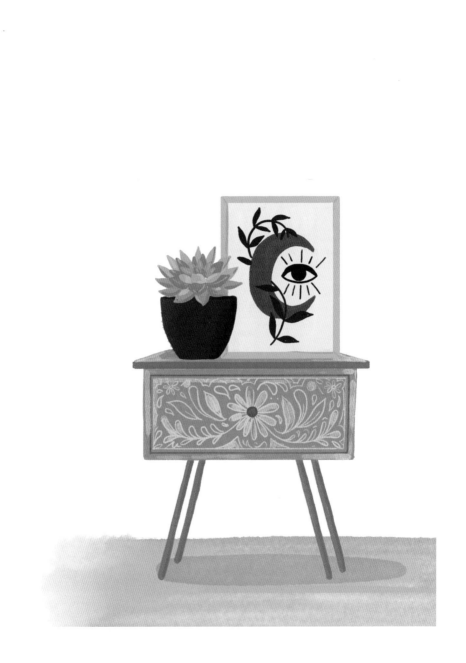

Let's move this into the bedroom.

This is the room where relaxation and a soothing environment are on the top of the must-have list when it comes to decorating. Since you may not get as big an audience of plant appreciators through here as you would your living room (but hey, if you do, no judgment), this is a space where the plants you nurture should be for your well-being, body and mind.

When we think about the primary purpose of the bedroom, we usually land on the idea of "rest." However you achieve that rest (again, no judgment) is an individual decision, but ultimately you come to this room for "sore labour's bath, balm of hurt minds"—if you don't mind a little Shakespeare.

But the bedroom is also a space of intimate self-expression. Our youthful bedrooms were such vivid expressions of ourselves. Don't try to pretend you didn't have a boy band or swimsuit model poster on your wall. Or were you one of those cutesy types with a ruffled counterpane, or did you have endless sports memorabilia? As we hone our maturity, we somehow get the idea that the way to achieve rest is to be so unbearably dull that you have to pass out. Leaving aside the few free-expression souls with tapestries and candles, most adults have bedrooms that are white. Or beige. Or gray. Bed, nightstand, dresser, piles of clothes you were too lazy to hang up or wash, books you're totally going to read soon, a picture of your mom. Some throw pillows if you're fancy.

Is this really what we need to achieve a true respite from our day's labor?

No matter your personal style, houseplants can create a relaxing sanctuary that helps you unwind, breathe better, and feel truly at home.

Start with a Deep Breath: Succulents

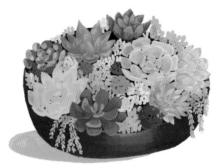

Breathe in. And slowly breathe out. There, don't you feel better already? By now you should know that many houseplants contribute positively to your welfare by cleaning the air, absorbing toxic chemical by-products of building and cleaning so you don't have to breathe them in. Remember that NASA study on using houseplants as natural air filters? Yes, many of your favorite indoor plants are diligently removing nasty stuff from the air as they grow. No, this does not mean you should smoke in front of them. They are very impressionable.

There is a certain species of houseplants, however, that offers some extra nighttime atmospheric benefits: the succulents.

Most plants release oxygen through their respiration process all day, using light and sunshine to photosynthesize some food and then pumping unneeded oxygen back out into the air. When the light stops, they take a break. Some succulents, on the other hand, continue producing oxygen all night long, making them the perfect plants to support your sleep.

Top of that list is the **snake plant**, or sansevieria. Its stiff, spiky leaves with little serrated points along their edges stand straight up, earning them another common nickname: mother-in-law's tongue. Snake plants tend to be dark green with variegated patterns in lighter shades.

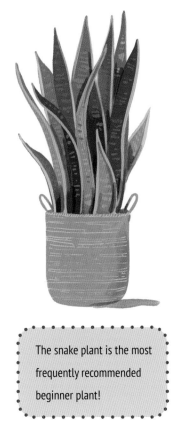

"That's my number-one choice for everyone, not just beginners," says Crystal Desi of Cactus Moon. "It thrives inside. The basic care is never water it unless the soil is completely dry. It's good for people who will be a little neglectful."

While the snake plant is super hardy, its low-stress needs aren't that different

The snake plant is the most frequently recommended beginner plant!

from more touchy succulents. Watering is where you need to be really careful. Use a fast-draining potting mix (a cactus potting soil mix is a good choice) and a pot with drainage holes.

"Trendy doesn't come with instructions," Desi says. "People will find something thrifting, but when you put your succulent in a cute little unicorn mug with no drainage holes, the poor plant has no chance."

She uses a ceramic drill bit to drill drainage holes in creative containers. If that's not your unicorn mug of tea, just get a proper plant pot. Not that a good pot is a guarantee of good plant parent behavior.

Here's a typical succulent newbie story of bad decisions: A customer told Desi he would keep his succulents inside and promised not to overwater. But a few weeks later, she got an SOS and a photo. "The plants had just been showered down, pots filled to the brim. The table they were on was holding water. And to dry them out quickly, he put them outside in direct sun. All the leaves had turned black."

Poor little succulents will get as bad a sunburn as you will if you forget sunscreen on a day at the beach. Don't take your succulent to the beach! In general, these plants want around six hours of light—but it's okay if it's artificial light. So if your bed-

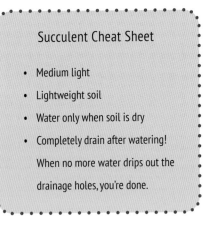

Succulent Cheat Sheet

- Medium light
- Lightweight soil
- Water only when soil is dry
- Completely drain after watering! When no more water drips out the drainage holes, you're done.

room lacks bright windows, you will still be helping your succulents grow when you stay up late reading your favorite book on houseplants.

A Few Favorite Succulents for Some Clean Air at Midnight:

- Jade plant, also called money plant or dollar plant, is known for its thick, juicy leaves, but it can also produce little white flowers in the winter. It brings you good luck!
- Burro's tail, or donkey's tail, grows brilliant-green, fleshy, droplet-shaped leaves in rows down a trailing stem. A great hanging plant for a tiny bedroom.
- String of pearls is a trailer like the burro's tail, only its "leaves" are tiny green globes scattered along a cascading stem.
- Haworthia is low-growing and small, a spiky cluster of thick, fleshy leaves that can feature white bumps or stripes (earning it the name zebra haworthia). A good bedside table companion.
- Hens and chicks (or sempervivum), another petite plant, is a very popular and varied succulent known for propagating as rapidly as any barnyard fowl. The "mother" plant, a frosty rosette, produces smaller offshoot "chicks" in clusters around it.
- Echeveria looks very similar to hens and chicks—a rosette of thick leaves. Its varieties are dazzling in color, from the pale-green Mexican snowball to the purple dusty rose to the silvery ghost echeveria.

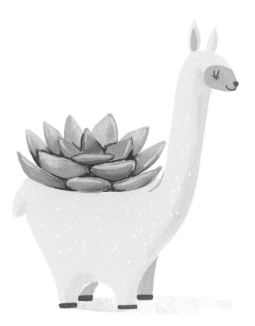

There are dozens more easy-to-find and gorgeous options. But from the dramatic snake plant to the dainty echeveria, please follow Desi's advice on how to meet your succulent's needs: "Just say something nice and walk along."

Your succulent will answer with better night air for peaceful sleep, so you wake rested and ready to focus back in on your bedroom style and decor.

Orchids Are the New Throw Pillows

It's not that they're not cuddly, but when it comes to a natural beauty to soothe the eye and create a spa atmosphere of tranquillity, a faux-fur cushion isn't really doing the job, is it? Instead, consider filling your space with the luxe brilliance of an orchid collection—even your most minimalist decor will come to life if you grace your windowsill with vivid purple blooms.

Orchids require attention and patience. On the one hand, orchids are specific about their needs, touchy when those needs are violated, and consult only themselves about when they feel like blooming. On the other hand, they are remarkably easy to maintain if you follow their rules and they bloom for as long as twelve weeks at a time. Mary Beth Shaddix of Maple Valley Nursery often tells would-be plant parents that while "everything has a life cycle, orchids come as close to a permanent plastic plant as anything."

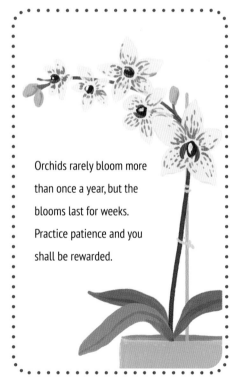

Orchids rarely bloom more than once a year, but the blooms last for weeks. Practice patience and you shall be rewarded.

If you've ever owned a cat, you know what you're in for with an orchid.

This is a tropical plant, so before you bring home your orchid, check your space to see if you're up for providing a lifestyle to which it is accustomed. Orchids need sun. If your bedroom is a dark and unlit zone, sorry, but move on to the next section. However, they can't take direct sun, so if your windowsill is drenched in hot light all day, put a cat there instead.

The rest is up to you—will you respect the law of the orchid?

1. No wet roots. Who wants to stew in a damp mess? Don't pack an orchid with heavy soil or moss. Give those roots good air circulation. Orchids should be potted in a specialty orchid mixture, which is probably going to include a loose bark. Orchid pots have big drainage slits so water runs right through.

2. Humidity is good for the skin and your orchid. During dry seasons and in dry climates, leave a tray of wet pebbles under your orchid pot. The water will evaporate around your tropical friend—and maybe even offer a little soothing humid air for you.

3. A little drought is a good thing—no puddles in the orchid pot. Wait until that pot is completely dried out—so dry you think it can't possibly survive—and then give it a good shower. Literally. Shaddix says to put orchids right under the shower head for watering—they love it! Other

orchid lovers swear by the ice-cube-in-the-pot trick for a slow, continuous dampness as the ice melts.

4. Fertilize both right before and right after your orchid blooms. As soon as buds start to form on a flower stalk, that's a good time to add a little extra fertilizing energy. Flowers are hard work, and your orchid deserves the support.

5. If you screw up, don't go to bed angry. Spot the signs of your misdeeds and apologize. Yellowing leaves (we're not talking about the old leaves at the base of the plant, which will yellow and die naturally, but all of the plant's poor leaves) might mean it's getting too much direct light, or is too chilly, or has rotting wet roots. If the leaves are black, that's probably a fungal infection—cut those leaves off and spray with fungicide.

It may take some time and even a failure or two to perfectly meet your orchid's needs. That's okay. Relationships take work. Do it right and you'll be rewarded with an annual bloom of rare perfection.

There are too many orchid varieties, including dozens of rare, wild species, to list without boring you to tears, but here a few that are relatively easy to track down:

- Moth orchid (Phalaenopsis) is probably the most commonly sold and photographed, with elegant, colorful blooms.

- Cattleya orchid produces big ruffled flowers in bright
  whites, yellows, pinks, and purples. Some varieties
  even offer a lovely fragrance.
- Lady of the night (Brassavola) is a great choice for
  a beginner because it's undemanding and doesn't
  mind if you forget to water. Its flowers are small
  and plain white but they bloom a lot, all year round.
  It's a lovely bedroom choice because it releases a
  marvelous fragrance only at night, to sweeten your
  dreams.
- Oncidium orchids bloom with tons of flowers, and
  the dozens of varieties will give you your choice
  of color and fragrance, like the Sharry Baby, or
  chocolate orchid, if you want your bedroom to smell
  like Willy Wonka's chocolate factory.

Bromeliads are the orchid's more chill companions. They like a lot of the same stuff but will be a little more relaxed about your burgeoning plant-care capabilities. Yes, they can flower periodically, pushing out long-stalked, wild-looking blooms in purples and pinks. But their day-to-day wear is also fabulous, ranging from the more traditional green-leaf look to red and orange foliage reminiscent of a rooster on the prowl.

Let's look at the basics of plant care: light, soil, water, food.

Bromeliads are going to want bright light, but will burn in too much direct light. Yellowing leaves indicate a sunburn, while dark-green leaves might be the bromeliad equivalent of pasty skin that needs more sunshine.

Even though bromeliads are, like orchids, epiphytes (most epiphytes, or air plants, attach to other plants or trees to steal their nutrients or har-vest energy straight from the sun and air), they don't mind getting their roots dirty. Plant them in a fast-draining soil and pot.

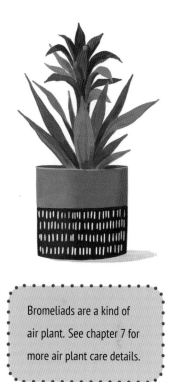

Water thoroughly, but watch out for bromeliad varieties that have a cup-shaped center among the leaves, where water can collect. Outside, those cups keep your plant moisturized through dry spells. Inside, that water can build up salts that need to be cleaned out. Only water the soil. And, if your climate is very dry, add a little humidity by misting the soil, moving your bromeliad to a more humid room, or setting it on a tray of pebbles and water.

Bromeliads are a kind of air plant. See chapter 7 for more air plant care details.

Fertilize when your bromeliad is working on growing a flower or an off-shoot. Reward that effort.

Some bromeliads to consider:

- Guzmania is that bromeliad you've probably seen in any plant or flower store. Its flower bract—that central stalk of leaves—shows up in dramatic reds, oranges, yellows, and pinks.

- Vriesea look really far-out. They start off fine with those typical bromeliad spiky green leaves. Then they pop out a sword of a flower bract in bright colors, with little blooms appearing along the edges. This flower lasts for months.
- Cryptanthus would be lovable for their leaf patterns—white-and-green chevrons, pink and red edges—even if they didn't produce wild pink-and-purple blooms. They only bloom once, though, so make sure you appreciate the moment!

A word about propagating (this is the "bedroom" chapter, after all): this is kind of a big deal when you're raising bromeliads. After a brief brilliant flowering comes to an end, the whole plant begins to fade away and die. Not all species die after flowering, but enough do to make it something to consider when you're raising bromeliads. Don't worry—this is their natural life process, like a butterfly dying after laying its eggs.

But, like that butterfly, the bromeliad reproduces before it dies. Some varieties produce delightfully named "pups," or offshoots, of new plants around the base of the parent plant. They can be parted from the parent plant when it begins to die and then repotted by nestling the pup in soil until it starts to root. Or just cut away the dead parent plant. Other bromeliads create new plants on shoots that grow along the soil surface that can similarly be repotted or, if you have the space, can grow into quite a collection of plants. You've now grown a bromeliad family in the privacy of your own bedroom!

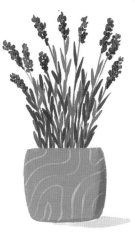

SET THE MOOD

You've set the atmosphere—rich, oxygenated air thanks to your succulents. You've set the tone—delicate beauty from your patiently tended orchids and bromeliads. Now how about a little scent therapy to take things to the next level?

Flowering plants with heady scents to attract pollinating insects typically do better out of doors with access to bright sun, but there are a few indoor successes that might help create aromas that complement your personal oasis.

Lavender's association with calm and sleep won't surprise you—lavender scent is found in all kinds of relaxation tonics, from baby wash to lotions to those ubiquitous essential oils. The real thing, the lavender plant, surpasses its own hype: vivid purple stalks of tiny flowers with an alluring woodsy, astringent scent.

Sunshine and lots of it is the key to a thriving indoor lavender bush. Here's a plant that actually likes direct sun. It doesn't need much water, either. It likes a little drought, so water only when the soil is bone-dry and make sure you keep the water off its perfumed leaves. It likes a compact growing space that gives its root ball only an inch or two of extra growing space, so no big pots.

When your lavender blooms, you can prune its flowers and dry them for cooking or making homemade sachets to spread its fragrance to other spaces.

May your dreams be populated with visits to Provence's sunny lavender fields.

Lavender is great when all you want is a good night's sleep, but we're adults here, so let's talk about those nights when you're not looking to nod off right away. Why not fill the air with the heady and romantic scent of gardenia?

Gardenias were reportedly Sigmund Freud's favorite flower. Let that sink in for a moment.

Growing gardenias indoors will take some effort, but the reward is that unforgettable and penetrating gardenia scent, the rich, evocative, almost lurid odor of Gilded Age buttonholes or Billie Holiday's floral crown. This is a warm-climate plant—the biggest threat to its success is cold temperatures, so you need to make sure you can provide more warmth than just your charming personality. Keep the room temperature above sixty degrees (if you're keeping your gardenia on a windowsill, check that temp carefully, since cold outside air can seep in) and try adding some humidity. Chilly gardenias will drop their flower buds just to punish you.

Gardenias are members of the coffee plant family (will that keep you awake at night?) and like an acidic potting soil—there are specialty varieties for gardenias or rhododendrons—with good drainage. Water regularly. This is not a snake plant that you can neglect for a few weeks. The gardenia relationship is definitely high maintenance. It knows what it wants and it's not afraid to ask for it. Pay it the proper worshipful attention and you will earn the crisp white blossoms that speak of moonlit nights and sultry breezes.

WORK FOR IT

One thing you may have noticed about the plants suggested in this chapter: with the exception of the super simple snake plant, these are not the most low-maintenance plants to get involved with. There's a reason for that: your own mental well-being.

Interacting with nature lowers stress and anxiety. One study from Japan measured blood pressure and heart rate before and after spending time in a forest, and found that the forest environment had a positive impact on overall health. But while walking in the woods is nice, for most of us it's a little impractical on a daily basis. We spend our lives indoors, so to take care of ourselves, we need to take a little of that outside in and bring nature to us. Even your littlest succulent has the power to soothe your nervous system.

Take time to pay attention to your plants: Do they need watering? Are they outgrowing their pots? Are they free from pests? How's the sunshine? In so doing, you are also taking time to pay attention to yourself. Slow, repetitive actions are commonly used in meditation techniques, which makes plant care a form of meditation.

Caring for plants, especially if you build up a good-sized collection, can take time and patience, and even some humility when you realize that as smart and capable as you are, you may not always be successful in raising that little green thing.

Mary Beth Shaddix encourages plant owners to give themselves a break—it doesn't always work out. "People will default to 'I can't do that'

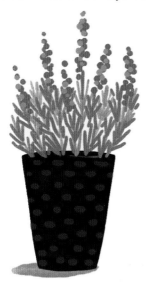

after they kill one plant. Sometimes you have to kill two or three plants before you learn what they love."

If your first effort at growing succulents or orchids is unsuccessful, don't take it as a personal failure. Learn from your mistakes, and also learn that some plants were just not meant to be. This lesson may be as valuable for easing your psyche as owning an indoor plant is.

Give yourself a break. Give your plant some love. Relax.

Now I Lay Me Down to Sleep

After a day of rigorous plant parenting, you can do no better than to follow the example of the **prayer plant** and fold your hands to rest when the day is done.

During the day, the prayer plant's wide, flat leaves show off feathery patterns of dark and light green, with red stems and underleaves for a dramatic appearance. But when the sun sets, the prayer plant's leaves fold inward like praying hands (guess how it got its name).

Here's the prayer plant care catechism:

1. No direct sunshine, but give your prayer plant plenty of light, especially in darker winter months.
2. Soil (preferably acidic) should drain well, no swampy roots.
3. But water frequently, especially during warmer months—unlike a lot of plants we've talked about in this chapter, you don't want to let the prayer plant completely dry out. Not too wet. Not too dry. Juuust right.
4. Mix that water with some diluted fertilizer every couple of weeks during the warmer months.
5. Mist at least once a week with warm water to give it that humid air it prefers.

Close up your leaves, rest well, and get ready to tackle tomorrow's indoor gardening projects.

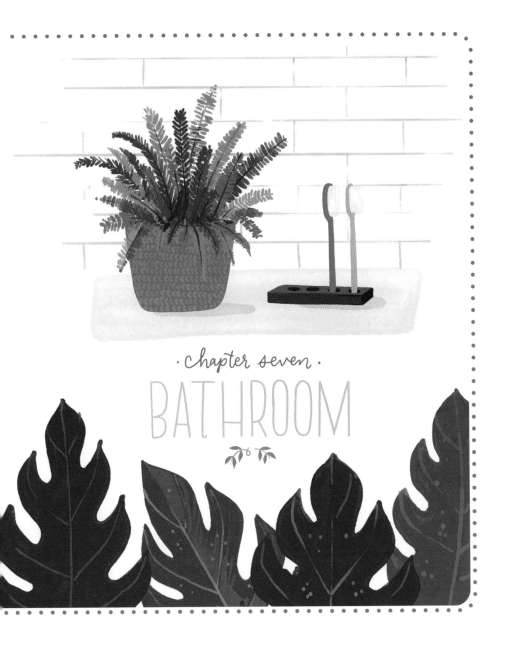

· chapter seven ·

BATHROOM

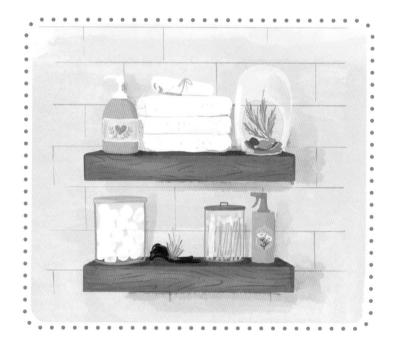

L et's be honest—this is a room where function rates pretty high over fashion. You can (barely) survive without matching hand towels, but there are certain elements to this space you just don't want to do without: toilet, sink (please tell us you wash your hands), shower/bath.

Still, there's no reason you can't dress up these essentials with some fancy touches. Your bathroom can be just as stylish, green, and fresh feeling as any other room of your house. Perhaps even more so, because of its unique environment.

For one thing, bathrooms are humid. Finally, after all the tropical plants listed in previous chapters exhorting you to give them the humid air they were born for, you've found a space guaranteed to make them happy. All of your long, hot showers and soothing baths, and even hand-washings, are a tropical plant's dream.

The trickiest thing about bathrooms can be their small size. Bathrooms are often among the more compact spaces in a home, unless you happen to live in a luxury hotel. Displaying your houseplants there can require a little creativity. You're not Tarzan; you don't want to wade through a jungle to go potty. Hanging plants, small plants, and plants that lend themselves to space-saving presentation are the friends of the restroom.

Let's start with air plants, plants that literally require no other display element than air itself.

Airing Out the Privy

Air plants, properly known as tillandsia, are having a moment, and there's no reason you can't be a part of it. Often confused with succulents, air plants are actually part of the bromeliad family, epiphytes that do not require—and will not grow in—soil. They thrive on air, light, and water, feeding themselves on photosynthesis alone. One has to admire their self-sufficiency. But one also has to care for them properly. They are unusual looking and more stubbornly independent, but they are still living beings that deserve TLC from time to time.

Ryan and Meriel Lesseig are husband-and-wife co-owners of Air Plant Design Studio, a national supplier of both common and hard-to-find air plants. Reminding people to love their air plants is step one of their jobs. As Meriel sometimes has to tell her customers: "Just because they are a lower-maintenance plant, they don't need *zero* maintenance!"

This is a lesson they teach customers who purchase air plants as gifts and leave them packed in a box for days or even weeks before presenting what will turn out to be a dead plant by that time. Ryan says one of their customers was upset when she learned air plants are not plastic—she wanted something to look at, not to care for.

But you do want to care for your air plant. Here's how:

The Lesseigs start by encouraging you to pick an air plant that suits your climate. There are two categories of air plants: xeric and mesic. Xeric tillandsias tend to be silvery in color thanks to "trichomes," which look little silver hairs covering the leaves but are actually tiny cups that gather water from the air for the plant to absorb. They hail from arid zones and survive harsher conditions with less rainfall and brighter sunlight. Dry climates and drier seasons might suit them best. Mesic tillandsias are rain forest natives, greener and happier with indirect light and wetter surroundings—be prepared to give these guys a little extra climate care if your environment doesn't lend itself to humidity.

Air plant experts like the Lesseigs offer lots of varieties of tillandsia, both the popular types and more expensive and rare plants. They even have special imports from South America, native land to many air plants. There are more than six hundred types of tillandsia in the world. You can surely find one or two to suit you and your bathroom needs. Get ready for a list of Latin names; air plants shun cutesy nicknames.

Tillandsia ionantha is a favorite for first-timers because it's relatively cheap, easy to come by, and can take a little more abuse than other plants. Small and compact, with silvery-green leaves, they blush bright pink before producing a light purple flower.

Tillandsia scaposa, sometimes known as *Tillandsia kolbii*, has a similar look, a cluster of hairy-looking leaves that turn pink and red before flowering. These can grow in a tight bunch, so be sure to shake out water carefully.

Tillandsia xerographica is very popular but more expensive and difficult to find because it's a protected species, meaning it takes a special permit to distribute. That doesn't stop it from showing up on Pinterest and Instagram on a regular basis, as it likes to show off its large, cushiony, silver style. This is a xeric variety, so it can handle lots of light and less water. **Tillandsia gardneri** has a similar look and needs, but with feathery leaves fountaining up from the center.

Tillandsia funkiana is as funky as you might expect. It doesn't grow in a tight cluster like many air plants. Its leaves grow along an extended stem, like a pine branch. The stem can twist or grow straight, ending in a flamboyant orange-red flower beloved of hummingbirds. Remember these are bromeliads—they produce lots of pups, or offshoots, along the stem.

The basics of air-plant care are the same as that of any other plant: light, air, and water.

Let there be light! While most air plants can't handle full hot sun, they do need plenty of light to keep themselves going. Place them near a window, but not in the direct glare of sunshine. If your bathroom is of the windowless-interior-tornado-shelter variety, the artificial glare of your light fixtures will work, as long as you keep then switched on for enough hours of the day to mimic natural daylight.

Wetter is better. But not that wet. Air plants like to suck moisture out of humid air, which makes the damp air from your daily showers a delight for this plant family. "The biggest loss to air plants is overwatering," Ryan says. "When the plant's color dulls and the leaves curl in a bit and look more concave, that means it's getting dehydrated and closing its leaves up to collect more moisture. Water once or twice a week, depending on the environment. Over time, you can start to tell when a plant wants water."

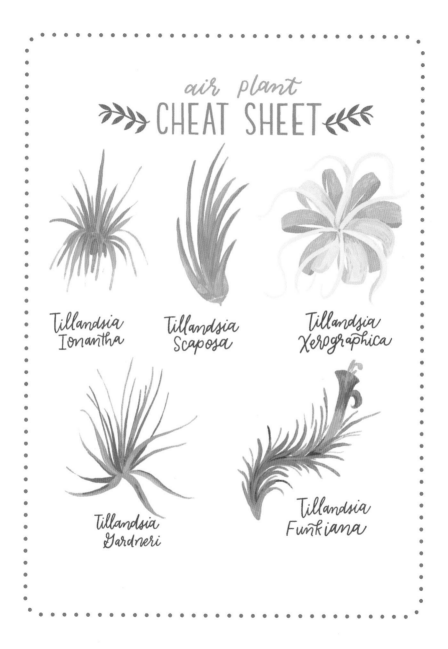

air plant
CHEAT SHEET

Tillandsia
Ionantha

Tillandsia
Scaposa

Tillandsia
Xerographica

Tillandsia
Gardneri

Tillandsia
Funkiana

When you need to water your air plant, submerge it in a bowl or sinkful of room-temperature water and let it soak for ten to twenty minutes, but not longer. You can also try repeatedly dunking your plant in water instead of soaking. With either method, make sure to shake off any extra water and let the plant dry completely before returning it to its proper setting—water left sitting on the plant can cause it to rot. And if your air plant looks sad and dry between waterings, especially in dry seasons or climates, a little light misting will help.

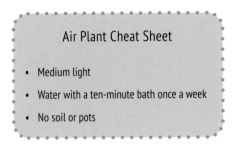

Air Plant Cheat Sheet

- Medium light
- Water with a ten-minute bath once a week
- No soil or pots

Air—it's in the name. It shouldn't come as a surprise that air plants need air. Specifically, they need good air circulation to constantly refresh their space. Enclosed containers like terrariums are better suited for plastic plants. Keep your air plant out in the open. Just remember that if it's near an air vent, it may dry out faster and need watering more often.

It's not only the typically more humid air of the bathroom that makes air plants so suited to this room—they are also well adapted to the complications of fitting houseplants into an already tight space. No pots allowed, no counter space or floor space clutter—these guys do well tucked into tiny corners and even displayed on walls or as hanging ornaments.

"You can display them in such a wide variety of places and still get good air circulation," says Meriel. For the home, she suggests a few popular display techniques that take advantage of the air plant's small size and disdain for convention:

Bathroom

- Vertical living walls can hold lots of air plants without taking up any of that precious counter space. Create a frame of chicken wire or crosshatch wire and use a fine wire or even a paper clip bent around your air plants to secure them to the chicken wire. Xeric air plants like xerographica will be especially attractive in this setting.

- Mixed with other accents, like balls or pinecones, in a centerpiece or a wooden bowl, air plants give a unique textural variety to the look.

- Since air plants are soil-free and dry, you can set them on a shelf without worrying about drainage or dirt; nestle them among magazines, lotion bottles, or other bathroom knickknacks to create an eye-catching display.

- Glue or set a smaller air plant in a shell or a sea urchin, on a piece of wood, or in a tea light holder. These are all great to suspend from fishing twine for an airy, light hanging plant to fill even the highest levels of your bathroom space. Using glue does come with a few complications, however. Be sure to use a plant-safe glue (most experts recommend the brand E6000); dab only a small amount on the plant's base, not its leaves; and be prepared to reglue after watering.

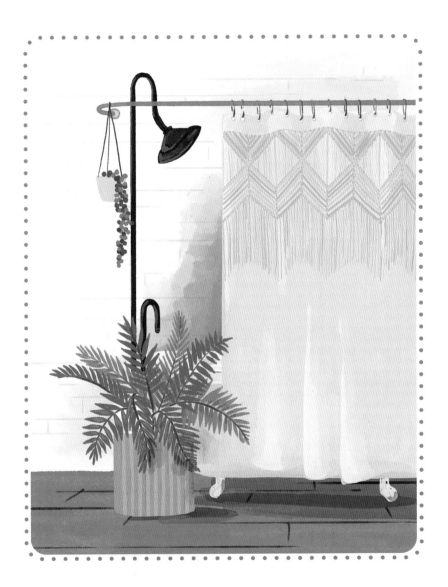

Thinking of You Frondly

Getting the hang of air plants but looking for something a little more traditional leafy-look for your personal spa? **Ferns** are your new friends. Ferns have been a popular space filler for homes, offices, doctors' lounges, and talk show host sets for decades.

Julie Bawden-Davis of HealthyHouseplants.com puts ferns firmly in the middle-maintenance category. This is not a species you can neglect or only visit when you remember, but it hasn't got the temperamental specificity of a truly difficult plant. You'll want to be on a schedule with fern care and thoughtful about choosing its rightful place in your house.

"A fern shouldn't dry out," says Bawden-Davis. "You can lose half the plant from just one time it dries out. It doesn't like that and it doesn't like dry air." Sounds like an ideal candidate for a powder room plant, right? It has the most humid air in the house and is a place you're guaranteed to visit regularly.

There are more than twelve thousand species of fern, the most ancient of the world's plants, so it should be easy to select your favorite, but there are a limited number that you can both readily obtain and readily tend indoors. These indoor species are largely tropical, so keeping them happy means keeping them in that tropical frame of mind. No, don't give them a mai tai, give them moisture.

(PS: If you're one of those people who can't stand the word "moist," you may want to pick a different houseplant.)

Moist . . . air. If you bathe daily, you will have some nice humid bathroom air. If you live in a particularly dry climate or it's a dry time of year, you can up the moisture level by giving that fern a spritz of water or keeping that oft-mentioned tray of damp pebbles in its vicinity. "Ferns transpire, releasing moisture into the air. When the air is more moist, they transpire less, so they're less likely to dry out," Bawden-Davis says.

Moist . . . soil. You have already read about succulents and cacti and other plants that like to dry out between waterings. Not so the fern. It likes to live in damp soil. Picture the jungle detritus where ferns grow wild and you'll get the idea. Damp doesn't mean soggy, though—soil should feel slightly wet to the touch, but not dripping or pooling in the bottom of the pot. Pick a soil that drains well but retains water; a soil that includes peat moss would be a good choice. Set up a weekly watering schedule to keep that fern moist.

Ferns will need light as well as humidity, but not direct sunlight. This is definitely a plant for a bathroom with a window. Ferns are used to feeding on the slowly rotting plant material of a forest floor, so fertilize gently. A slow-release fertilizer or diluted liquid formula will serve them best.

Here are some of our favorite fronded friends:

A **Boston fern** is more rarely called sword fern for the shape of its draping fronds. This is probably what you think of when you picture a fern, a plant with its long, arching fronds frilly with small finger-shaped leaves on each side creating a regular serrated pattern. It's not called "Boston" fern for any interesting reason; it was just found in a plant shipment from Florida to Boston in the nineteenth century and named for its location, not its accent. Boston fern is one of the easier members of the fern family, being able to handle a less rigorous watering schedule. It may take some time to determine the precise environment it needs in your home, but it will let you know if there's not enough humidity by turning yellow and dropping its leaves.

Some people like to cut back old growth as it starts to get overwhelmed by newer leaves, turning yellow and dry. Clip the old leaves off near the base to give new leaves—which start as tight, fuzzy curls—space to unfurl.

Notably, this familiar frond was one of the lucky few featured in the NASA study on plants that clean air. This guy will filter formaldehyde, xylene, and toluene (all toxic chemicals) from the air. A trait that's especially appreciated in a plant occupying the close quarters of the bathroom. Ahem.

Asparagus fern: This is the thing with feathers. It's not even a real fern (it's part of the lily family), it's just hoping to be thought of as such. Light, lacy foliage that looks like Muppet hair tops long, green stems that look like an asparagus stalk, but with sharp barbs. Approach with care, outside and in—just because it's called "asparagus" doesn't mean you can eat it! The

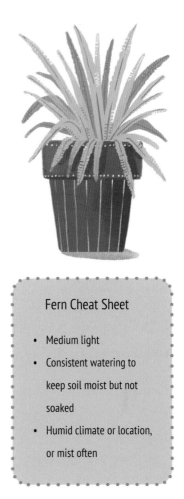

Fern Cheat Sheet

- Medium light
- Consistent watering to keep soil moist but not soaked
- Humid climate or location, or mist often

greens, flowers, and berries are all toxic to you and your pets. It needs potting soil that drains well, and it is best kept in indirect light. Humidity is key to a happy asparagus fern, which will dry up and turn brown without sufficient moisture. You may think it's dead, but it just needs more water! Mist it, let it hop in the shower with you, and maybe invest in one of those humidity trays. It doesn't need repotting often, preferring a snug-fitting (but draining) container. Trim it back regularly to make it bushier and denser.

Maidenhair fern: Oddly, this fern looks less like hair than the asparagus fern, featuring petal- or fan-shaped leaves scattered daintily along its fronds. That's because its name isn't a reference to its looks (or marital status). The Latin name of one variety, *Adiantum capillus-veneris*, very loosely translates into "unwetted Venus's hair" (Venus being the original maiden, and "unwetted" coming from the way water rolls off the leaves as easily as off a duck's back, as they say). The cuteness of the name is now shared with all *Adiantum* types. It has a prettiness that earns its name, however, and a list of delicate needs. Don't expose its modesty to bright light or sun; side glances of daylight will do. It droops without enough humidity and wilts without proper watering. A schedule won't suffice; you'll have to check how it's feeling frequently. It will turn brown or cast aside its leaves when it's unhappy; keep it slightly wet at all times. Julie Bawden-Davis calls the maidenhair fern the "queen of all pickiness." Approach with chivalry and be prepared to make a serious commitment.

Even though a thriving fern will be a bushy masterpiece of wild fronds, it doesn't have to be a big space suck in pocket-size square footage. Ferns look gorgeous as hanging plants. Those long branches of tiny leaves fan out over the pot rim for a classic but elegant look.

Hanging Gardens

Hanging plants are a great way to fit some foliage into compact corners of your home. Using that vertical space effectively can even make the room feel bigger, and including some aerial green beauty will transform it from utilitarian to enjoyable.

How to hang a plant? Get out your ladder and your drill, because you're going to need to attach a hook to the ceiling or wall. It is not considered rude to ask how much your plant weighs; in fact, we encourage it. Make sure to include pot weight as well, and select a hook designed to support that weight. Next, check the background structure for the location where you intend to drill the hole for a hook. Thin plaster or drywall will simply crumble, and no one wants to come home to a sad pile of fern, shattered pot, and drywall beneath a hole in your ceiling. Drill into a wall stud or sturdy cabinet, just as you would for a heavy picture frame.

Of course, not everyone wants to drill, baby, drill. Especially not your landlord. You can still enjoy the hanging plant look, just with a bit more inventiveness. Trailing stems look wonderful tumbling down from a high shelf or even from your shower caddy. Small, light plants, including air plants, can be suspended from a light fixture with a bit of clear fishing line. Wall sconces—whether specifically designed to hold plants or modified from a candle or light sconce—can make a smaller statement on bathroom walls.

So what else will hold its head high without pulling down your plaster? How about an old-fashioned coatrack? Stand it in a corner and hang a different plant from each arm, and you'll have a green tree of plant life taking up only a small space. Curtain rods—even your shower curtain rod—stretched across a wall will hold several plants at a time (though, again, make sure you know what kind of solid scaffolding hangs out behind your attractive wall paint choices). Or how about your towel rack?

There is a multitude of plants suited to be displayed in hanging baskets or attached to wall sconces. In addition to ferns, here are few other options that look particularly unique and dazzling dripping from the heights of your bathroom:

String of pearls is so odd looking, you will think you have borrowed it from an alien planet. It looks like you have strung a collection of green peas on a string (it's not anything like a pea, however, as it is definitely toxic to you and to pets if eaten), and as it grows it will dangle as much as two feet over the edge of your hanging pot. String of pearls is a succulent, and each bead is actually a thick, juicy spherical leaf—this is the plant's clever water storage solution. You'll know it's thirsty when the beads

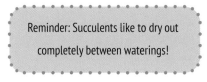

Reminder: Succulents like to dry out completely between waterings!

start to lose their plump roundness. Check back in chapter 6 for some reminders on how to grow succulents. String of pearls is an African desert plant in origin, and it's not looking for tropical climes. It needs a light, fast-draining soil and pot, and should be watered only when it's dry. Don't let it stand in soggy roots, and the natural humidity of a bathroom should be the limit of humidity you offer it. It's generally fairly easy to care for, as succulents go. Keep its environment stable and give it good air circulation.

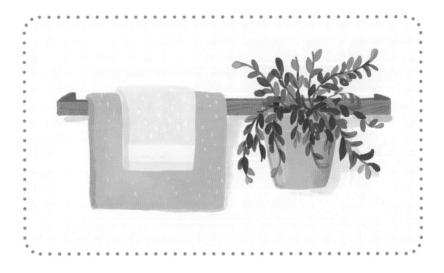

Goldfish plants have a similarly cool name and unique look, named as they are for the profusion of orange flowers that look like a school of gulping goldfish has taken over your nice houseplant. Go fish. Goldfish plants make wonderful hanging plants, with stems of small green leaves and orange flowers cascading down from the pot. This is a tropical plant, so unlike the string of pearls, it will gobble up any extra humidity in your bathroom. No direct light for this one, but it does need water, preferring a lightweight soil that is always a bit damp. *Damp*, not soggy. And keep the water off leaves and flowers to avoid fungus and mold. One reason this is a successful hanging plant is that it doesn't need a big pot to grow in, preferring to fit snugly without repotting too often. It doesn't flower year-round, but will flower more often if you keep it in a tight pot and good lighting. And unlike its namesake that sooner or later ends up, er, flushed, the goldfish plant can live a long time.

Many plants will grow well as hanging plants. Select them for the look you like, whether it's trailing stems or fuller branches. A few small adjustments to the usual guidelines for growing these particular houseplants can help make the experience a greater success:

1. Use a lighter-weight potting mix, heavier in perlite, so that wet soil isn't adding a risky extra pound to your planter.

2. Use a lighter-weight pot or basket. This is not the place for heavy terra-cotta or porcelain. Or if you're hanging an air plant, no pot required!

3. Water with caution. If you try to water a hanging plant in situ, be ready for a huge mess. This is fine if you happened to hang the plants over your bathtub, but otherwise you might want to remove them to a different location. To water properly, you need to make sure water runs out of the drainage holes—think carefully about whether you want that water dripping all over your walls and cabinets.

4. Water often. Hanging plants need watering a bit more frequently, since they're hanging out where that warm air tends to rise.

One final note: we've listed a lot of humidity-loving plants in this chapter, and while they all love the sultry air of a tropical night, be cautious about creating a jungle atmosphere in your own home. Humidifiers add moisture to your air, but please reserve them for your next head cold, not for your ferns. Keeping that level of moisture in an enclosed space will induce mold growth—in your walls, between your bathroom tiles, and even in your plant. Stick to misting the plants directly and taking advantage of the inevitable but shorter-term moisture from your showers.

Having completed your bathroom toilette (and we must say, you look fabulous), it's time to head into the office.

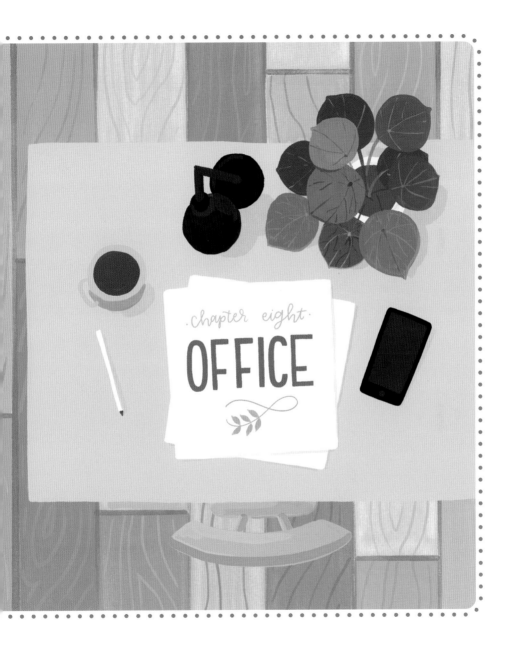

.chapter eight.

OFFICE

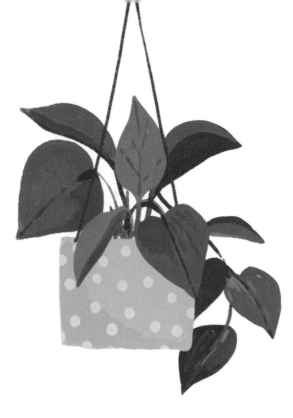

Hey, it's been nice hanging out at home with you, but if you're going to finance your burgeoning houseplant habit, you're going to have to get a job. Fear not: your plants will be fine from nine to five. Just give them a little extra focus (ficus?) when you get home. Quality thyme.

If you have a home office, the concern is moot. Your urban jungle can spread effortlessly from parlor to study. Even without work-from-home opportunities, however, you can enjoy plant life in your work life.

In fact, a good office plant will help reduce your stress and push you to greater productivity. Seriously! Companies are constantly trying to find ways to get better workers. For a while, the design trend of "lean" (that's fancy for barren, lifeless) decor held sway until a few studies reminded everyone that people tend not to work hard in the void. In fact, research has been telling corporations that the best way to keep a rat moving in the rat race is to give it a nice houseplant.

"Businesses want people to stay in their building, to attract people and keep them there. It's about creating environments that are warm and welcoming," says Matt Kostelnick of Ambius. "When you're inside of a building, you're taken away from a natural environment. Plants are one of the easiest ways to bring an aspect of nature back into a building."

The required office furnishings are hardly inspiring on their own. Desk. Chair. Computer. Phone. Feel energized? We didn't think so. Filling those plain walls and empty spaces with personal items can nudge the room toward a place where you feel comfortable. You could hang your college diploma on the wall, if you're one of those types. You could frame a picture of your mom, as long as her image reminds you of unconditional support, not questions about whether you're wasting that expensive college degree she paid for. But how much more fulfilling would it be to turn your view of the photocopier into a view of a philodendron?

"Imagine being in a room with all-white walls, nothing to stimulate you," Kostelnick says. "Plants make a place look higher-end, and help you differentiate yourself."

Whether you work for a giant, evil corporation or a do-gooder nonprofit, or just by yourself, all the research shows that a little plant life in the office space increases job satisfaction, concentration, and just *feeling* like the air quality is better. One study found that students hanging with houseplants were able to focus on work for longer, without feeling tired out by the intellectual rigor. A few other "productive plant" findings:

- People who work near plants had 15 percent more ideas than those who didn't (no word on whether they were good ideas).
- A plant placed near a computer caused the person using it to be 12 percent speedier.
- Reports of "a case of the Mondays" and "casually absent Fridays" dropped from 15 percent to 5 percent.

- Plants in elementary school classrooms led to improved grades for kids—don't you still want that A?

Of course, selecting a plant to share your desk could be as troublesome and time-consuming as hiring new staff, so we called in HR (that's the Houseplant Resources department) to suggest some questions for efficiently weeding through plant résumés for job compatibility:

What Is Your Ideal Work Environment?

When you look through lists of plants online or shelves of plants at garden stores, it can be difficult to distinguish which ones will thrive in your environment. Whether your office is at home or away, picking your plant should be as carefully approached as picking your staff.

Before you hit the local nursery, check your environment: What kind of work/life balance can your plant expect in this location? Are you blinded because your desk is located beside huge windows, or do you have to take frequent breaks just to go outside for a little sunshine? Match your office plants to your office lighting. Do you have to bundle up in a sweater in July because you sit under an AC vent, or do you swelter next to radiator? Find a plant that likes the temps in your work climate. Do you have a massive mahogany desk or a tiny cubicle? Pick a plant that is a size that fits in your work space. Most important question: Are you going to be an easy work companion for that plant?

"Consider what your office is like and how often you are going to be there," says Kostelnick. "Are you there every day? Are you going to take a three-week vacation? Pick something that is pretty low-maintenance. And I wouldn't bring in a ton of plants. Start small."

Are You a Self-Starter?

When you're thinking about desk companions, this is not the time to be experimenting with a complex calamondin orange tree. You need a plant that will support your efforts to stay focused and get the job done. The easy-to-grow category is the best bet.

Kostelnick recommends selecting an office plant from your earlier successes in houseplantery. Did your pothos smile upon you from your home coffee table? Put a pothos on your desk. Has that snake plant you forgot in your bedroom corner survived despite the odds? Try moving it next to the whiteboard to stimulate ideas.

What Are Your Plans for Growth?

Even the most low-maintenance plant requires some maintenance. When you're planning your plant decor, think through your plant care plans. Unless you're keeping a bag of potting soil in your filing cabinet and a watering can beside the copier, you'll need to carve out time and space for checking in on your plant's job satisfaction somewhat more often than your annual review. This can be a good thing for you, too. While office life can sometimes be boringly routine—no matter how passionate you are about your chosen career, let's not pretend sorting through your emails in the morning fills you with eternal joy—this can actually be an advantage for your plant.

Getting the watering schedule wrong for your plant is the quickest way to a houseplant exit interview. "People will assume more water is always better," says Kostelnick. "If the plant isn't doing well, they'll assume more water is needed. The plant doesn't drink itself to death, but roots also need air; if the roots can't breathe anymore, they drown."

The office, however, is a scheduled environment. Unlike the bedroom or the kitchen, which you may enter at odd times of the day, the office runs on routines. Put it on your calendar: Tuesday morning after the staff meeting, check to see if your plant's soil is ready for a bath.

To be clear, when we say "water," we mean water, not other liquid options. Your houseplant is not where you should dispose of this morning's cold coffee—or that beer you should not have during work hours. Think this is a silly thing to point out? "People stash things in plants all time," Kostelnick says. "It happens all the time. It's the hiding place—trash, wrappers, something you want to hide."

Please give your rubber plant love, not rubbish.

This is a hefty portfolio of plant-vantages to look through. Once you've carefully reviewed your applicants, it's time to start hiring.

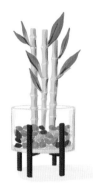

Entry-Level Position

You can do no better than to start with a **lucky bamboo**. This bundle of jointed, light-green stalks crowned by intermittent leaves is probably already familiar to you. It has graced many a desk or windowsill in its time, sometimes growing straight, sometimes manipulated into spirals or woven into interesting shapes. Like you, it has lied on its résumé to get the job (we know you're not really "proficient in Excel"): it's not really bamboo. Lucky bamboo, or *Dracaena sanderiana*, is actually related to the corn plant you encountered in chapter 3, and it's even easier to keep alive. Fit it snuggly into a cute pot and, as they say, just add water. Keep the water level about an inch deep above the roots and refresh it at least once a week to prevent bacteria from growing in the sit-

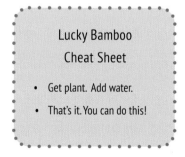

Lucky Bamboo
Cheat Sheet

- Get plant. Add water.
- That's it. You can do this!

ting water. If your tap water is high in chlorine, let it sit out overnight to evaporate before feeding it to your chemically sensitive bamboo. Potting soil will also work if you prefer that look. This dracaena doesn't need a ton of light and will burn in direct sun. It will grow toward the light, so rotate it regularly to maintain those straight, sturdy stalks. Trim excessive leaves and offshoots if it's getting too bushy or top-heavy.

Lucky bamboo will, of course, bring you good luck and great fortune. Bonus if you got it as a gift. Even if it was a gift to yourself.

A little bit of luck comes along with the **purple shamrock plant**, as well. It's popular around St. Patrick's Day, naturally, but unlike a lot of the behaviors that make you late to work on March 18 every year, it can be a perennial delight. Purple shamrock plant, aka black oxalis, is a garden pest when outside, but as an indoor plant, it works as a rare black or purple design contrast to the usual houseplant greenery. Its wine-colored leaflets are triangular, clustered in groups of three bending gracefully from a pale white stem. The leaves close in on their stems at night and reopen in daylight. The stems emerge from a bulb, a large rhizome that rests just under the soil. Oxalis won't want direct sun, so an interior space will work. Water well at first to get it going, but an established bulb doesn't benefit from frequent watering. After its summer growing season, it gets a little leggy looking, but trim it back closer to the bulb and it will regrow in the spring. It might even produce dainty pink flowers! While wishing on a shamrock won't get you a promotion, it will definitely improve your office mood to have a little Goth houseplant companion.

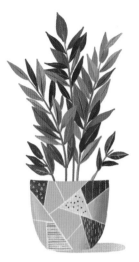

MIDDLE MANAGEMENT

A master of orderly design and straightforward care, the **ZZ plant** rewards those who show up and get the job done without too many fussy details. Its shiny green leaves are so neatly polished and arranged that its design is itself an invitation to dot i's and cross t's.

The ZZ plant is a tropical plant from Africa. It's on the NASA list of air-purifying plants, with a talent for removing the toxins xylene, toluene, and benzene from the air—a great contribution to the office team. We already reviewed ZZ plant watering in chapter 2, but let's circle back. To recap, water thoroughly until water flows through drainage holes. Then let it dry out completely. It traps this water in big, chunky rhizomes that look like potatoes—when these start to push against the pot, it's time for a bigger pot. No direct sunlight, but ZZ starts looking scraggly when it doesn't get enough light. Go with a medium level of exposure or lots of "unnatural" light. Those polished leaves will need dusting from time to time, too.

The ZZ plant also does well with a little neglect, so this is an ideal companion for when you're focusing on your career.

Sometimes work can feel like you're shuffling through life, so why not **schefflera** through it instead? Schefflera is, like ZZ, a tropical plant (from the northern East Asian islands) that looks good both as a small desk plant when you're just starting out and as a big floor plant when you're starting to feel like this might be a profession, not just a job. It's also called an umbrella plant after the look of its oval green leaves arching out from a central stalk.

Like the ZZ plant, the schefflera scorns overwatering. When you water (and make sure the pot drains completely), soak the soil and then let it dry out. It will let you know if it's been overwatered by dropping its leaves. If it's getting enough light—though not direct light—it can grow as high as six feet indoors, but prune it back if you like it smaller or if lack of light is making it little gangly. A good trim will encourage it to grow back leafy and luxuriant.

Schefflera Cheat Sheet

- Indirect light, not too bright
- Water when soil is dry and make sure even large pots (this plant can be a big guy) drain completely—no sitting water in the bottom of the pot

Executive Floor

Promotion! Having recognized the value and significance of incorporating a green theme in the work zone, you are ready to target more effective output: let's earn some money.

Yes, we know. You love your career and every day is so fulfilling. But we're guessing that career might be a little less fulfilling without the paycheck, so ask your houseplant, can you help me get rich? That's a little unlikely, but take a look at a few plants that might motivate your work-life achievement.

Fêng shui recommends harnessing a plant's energy to stir your own energies. As your plant prospers, so shall you. Placing a houseplant in the southeast section of your space, the "money area," enhances financial energy. Placing a houseplant in the east, the "health area," brings nourishing energy to keep your mind and ideas growing. Placing a houseplant in the south, the "fame area," fires your get-up-and-go. Placing a money tree in any of these corners is sure to bring you wealth, hopefully in both your personal vitality and your bank account. But which money tree?

Also known as the money plant, the lucky plant, the friendship tree, or *Crassula ovata*, the **jade plant** is a popular symbol of good fortune. It's also a relatively low-maintenance plant, another auspicious sign that it belongs in your office.

Jade is a name it has earned, its oval, fleshy green leaves reminiscent of the precious mineral. The leaves branch from a trunklike stem that, as the jade plant matures, looks like the finely drawn trees of a Japanese

painting. This is a succulent, so its pot and soil need
to drain well so it doesn't become a drain on your work
productivity. Water it thoroughly; drain it thoroughly;
resist watering again until
the soil is dried out. You
don't want to have to tell the

> Jade plants are so easy to propagate, you'll
> want to share with coworkers. Snip off
> a few leaves, set them on some potting
> soil, and keep that soil moist until you see
> baby plants start to develop along the cut
> edge. Those are new jade plants! More on
> propagation in chapter 9.

boss you were late with a report because you were busy mourning the
yellow leaves on your dying jade plant. Unlike many of the other office
plants profiled, this one needs lots of sun, even direct sun. If you're keeping it in a more secluded corner of your office, move it to a windowsill at
least once a week to soak up some rays. It won't need to be repotted often,
but refresh the soil every few years.

If you do your part well, you may be rewarded with tiny, white starlike
flowers, a different kind of symbol of success. Even if your bank account
doesn't reflect the tradition of jade plant's effect on financial prosperity,
take pride in the achievement of a healthy jade plant.

Here's where it gets confusing: Guiana chestnut is the **money tree**.
Seems like everybody's just trying to make a buck these days. This money
tree features a leaf pattern probably familiar to you from horse chestnut
trees common in American parks design. Its shiny leaves are arranged in
clusters of six sprouting from each stem. The tree is popularly sold as a
group of three or more trunks braided together to create a compact bushy
plant that fits nicely on a desk if you keep it pruned, or as a large floor

plant if you don't. Repotting will encourage it to get bigger fast, so keep the pot small if you favor the diminutive.

Give your money tree a medium amount of light and a really well-draining pot, because it likes to be watered a lot but can't tolerate staying soaked. Water when the top inch of soil is dry—that soil should be a rich potting soil, but one that drains fast, maybe even a cactus mix. Those lovely shiny leaves ought to be dusted regularly, and misting them during this process gives them a little extra humidity.

This is a hardy plant, but remember: the fêng shui benefits only come from healthy plants. Keep as close an eye on your money plant as Scrooge keeps on his money.

The **coin plant** is also known as the Chinese money plant. Yup, that's right, another one. And it's as different from the previous varieties as they are from each other. The coin plant is adorable, a little jewel of a plant, with circular (coin-shaped) green leaves on slender stems. It also goes by the names pancake plant and UFO plant after its leaf shape, or missionary plant, presumably a reference to its reputed travel history: a Norwegian missionary brought it home from China in the 1940s and shared cuttings with friends. It certainly figures frequently in Scandinavian interior design, a rounded green antidote to spare, simple furnishings.

Medium light works for this cutie (picture the light in a Norwegian winter and you'll get the idea). Direct sun will scorch it, while a little shade will sometimes encourage larger leaves. Give it good drainage, of course, so it can get nearly, but not entirely, dry between waterings. Those pancake leaves go limp when it needs watering. The leaves also need regular dusting, so misting it or giving it a hearty shower will help.

Whether this type of money plant will amplify your good fortune is debatable. It certainly didn't help that Norwegian missionary, who was kicked out of China, but with a plant this sweet decorating your work space, don't you already feel fortunate?

Whether your plants are money or not, a little extra green never hurt anyone, in your pocket or in a pot on your windowsill.

Let's Talk Bonus

Personal success, that loosely defined concept, comes in many forms. In the end, we decide it for ourselves. If success to you looks like wealth, fine. If it means serving your community, awesome. If it means time for family and friends, lovely. If it means a houseplant on your desk, bringing you cleaner air, greater productivity, reduced stress, and maybe even a little bit of luck, then that sounds like success to us.

We spend a lot of time in a work environment, and it can sometimes be hard for us to disconnect at the end of the day, turn off work brain and turn on Friday night brain. Can that affect your office plant?

"Sometimes people will not let go of their plants," says Matt Kostelnick. When his company is ready to trade out a plant past its prime in an office building, they can have a hard time prying it away from their customers. "If they've had a plant in their office for the last ten years, they've grown attached to it. It doesn't matter what it looks like. It could be dying. We'll want to replace it and they won't let us."

Of course, if when you should have been working you've instead spent a lot of time building a deep and complex relationship with your plant, then it would naturally be hard to separate. That, too, is kind of . . . different.

"People will talk about plants as though they actually have feelings," Kostelnick says. "I've heard of people talking *to* their plants."

We love houseplants, too, but please be aware that if you're talking to your plant and the plant talks back, it's time to step away and seek some human companionship instead. Use your houseplant as a conversation starter to build relationships with coworkers. Connect over coin plants. Bond over bamboo. Look around the office and you'll be able to spot the fellow plant people—they're the ones with smiles on their faces and vines trailing off their desks. Talk to them when you just can't stop thinking about whether it's time to dust the dracaena.

And if a coworker catches you talking to a plant, we recommend pretending you were really on a conference call: "Yeah, let's get to the root of this problem. I'll leaf through those spreadsheets and dig deep on the data."

CORNER OFFICE

The view from the top always looks good. Especially if it includes a houseplant.

At the highest executive level, you can afford to spend more time on a houseplant, right? Actual work? You've got people for that. Delegate and dig into some rewarding but high-maintenance flora, like the **nerve plant**. It took nerve to get to your position, brazening it out and acting confident even when you didn't feel it. You are so ready to handle a challenging task like raising a nerve plant, or Fittonia, named for nineteenth-century Irish botanists and sisters Elizabeth and Sarah Mary Fitton. You have to admire people with the chutzpah to name discoveries after themselves! It's also called a mosaic plant or painted net leaf for the intricate pattern of green interspersed with pink, red, or white veins on its leaves. A Peruvian native, the nerve plant is low-growing, rarely higher than six inches. This is a delicate, warmth-loving, humidity-demanding diva suited to trailing from small containers, hanging baskets, or terrariums. Provide indirect light only, so if your corner office has huge windows, move it away from the brightest rays. If your climate is dry, adding a tray full of wet pebbles will help increase humidity around your Fittonia. Mist regularly, but don't overwater, as it likes moist soil but not wet soil. It will shrivel and look pathetic if underwatered, and turn yellow if overwatered.

Yes, you could prove your CEO-worthiness with desk accessories like crystal plaques and preposterously expensive pens, but if you master indoor nerve plant care, you'll know there is no challenge you are incapable of meeting head-on. Name it after yourself, like the Fitton sisters.

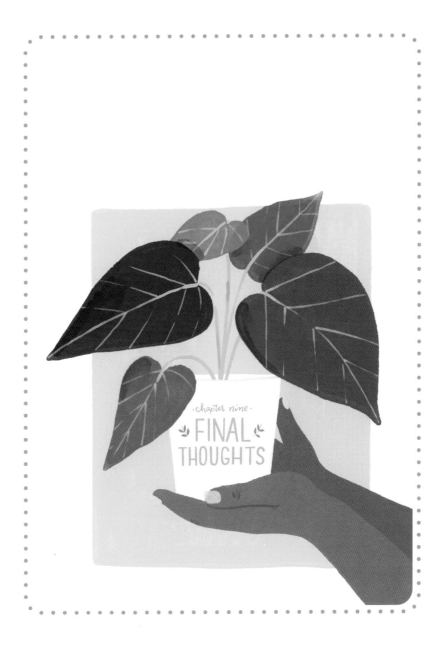

·chapter nine·

FINAL
THOUGHTS

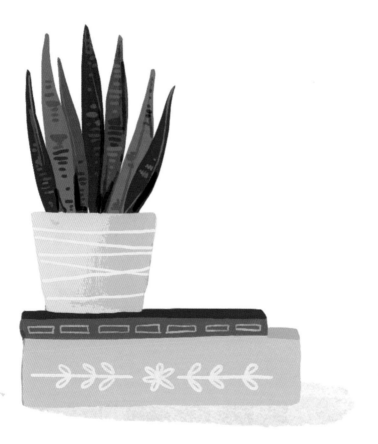

Time for a confession. This is not the definitive work on houseplants.

In truth, there is not a definitive work on houseplants. Houseplants are as infinitely varied and unique as any of your human companions. Whatever "facts" you gather about each houseplant you research, you should consider with care. The precise amount of water, the precise amount of sunshine, the perfect location will be yours to experiment with by old-fashioned trial and error. Take our recommendations as guidelines, not rules.

Whatever you learn from this or any book, your precious little plant is unique. As it grows, you'll grow alongside it as a plant parent until you, too, can say, "I get as much from my plant as it gets from me!" (But don't say this in public. You'll get some looks.)

The important thing is not to feel constrained or defeated by a plant. You can find a dozen variations in "the best way to care for houseplant X," and your most careful and dedicated efforts can still leave you with a dead houseplant. It's sad, but it's okay! Mary Beth Shaddix of Maple Valley Nursery says, "Everything has a life cycle." The important thing is that you keep trying. A green thumb isn't just something you're born with—it's a skill set you can nurture and grow over time.

It's common to get frustrated. You'll have bad days with your plants—the basil dried up; you forgot to mist your air plants; the ZZ was fine one day and dead the next—but there will be good days, too.

And can we let you in on a secret? There's no such thing as an "unkillable" plant. Even our plant experts copped to killing their fair share. As Julie Bawden-Davis of HealthyHouseplants.com says, "A lot of plant care is trial and error. Until you try something, you have no idea. It's all learning. Sometimes you have to kill some plants to learn."

See? No need to panic. If at first you don't succeed, plant again. Houseplants should be your reward for the challenges of modern life. Like you, it will not be perfect. But also like you, it will be beautiful.

Green Greenery?

What is your houseplant's carbon footprint? It seems like a strange question for a species without feet, but it's one that more and more plant owners are starting to ask. If you are raising a tropical plant in Minnesota or a cactus in Vermont or an areca palm in your New York apartment, you have probably realized that you are entertaining a friendly transplant.

Most purchased houseplants come from gardening centers or stores. Many of these get their supplies from large growers, whether grown in greenhouses or warm-climate fields, and like Americans themselves, most houseplants are immigrants. This has a medium to low environmental impact: gardening centers will get large plant orders delivered to them by a truck, which is certainly a polluter but also a fairly efficient way to move large quantities.

Online plant shopping gives you a greater array of plant options, including rarer and more unique varieties. Depending on how the plants are shipped to you (by truck? by plane?), this could have a higher environmental impact. However, this can also be an opportunity to get plants that have been sustainably grown and produced with low environmental impact, which is not always a guarantee with a gardening center. This is also an opportunity to help preserve species that are getting overrun or eliminated in the wild. Our air plant specialists, Ryan and Meriel Lesseig, import special endangered species from countries like Guatemala (this requires a permit!) and then can sell those plants, or propagate or hybridize them in their own nursery.

Don't overthink this: houseplants are not the major driver in human environmental damage. But thoughtfulness about from where you gather your urban jungle—grower, gardening center, or online store—does lead us to an additional option for fulfilling a mad houseplant passion.

Let's talk about propagation, baby.

The majority of houseplants you've encountered are so ready for a wild night of propagation. Reproducing a new baby plant from an existing mature plant doesn't even require a bottle of wine and some slow music. Just a little patience and a few tips.

Enough to Grow Around

Julie Bawden-Davis describes her first experience of plant ownership: "I started indoor gardening when I was seven. I actually found a coleus in the drugstore and brought it home. I kept it alive and started propagating it—I ended up with forty or fifty in my house!"

Coleus, also known as painted nettle or poor man's croton, is an outdoor border garden favorite popular since Victorian times, with bushy and delightfully varied foliage—varieties come in green, maroon, chartreuse, and red, and in all different patterns. But as seven-year-old Julie discovered, they also do well indoors. Part of the mint family (though not nearly as tasty), they can be reproduced from both seed and leaf cuttings.

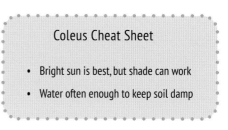

Coleus Cheat Sheet

• Bright sun is best, but shade can work
• Water often enough to keep soil damp

To propagate from seed, let the plant flower and go to seed and then harvest the results. You can grow a new coleus from the seeds, but be forewarned: the new plant may bear no resemblance to the parent plant. Almost all coleus plants are hybrids, a sophisticated word for "plant mutt." As with humans, genetic output is widely variable.

Propagating a coleus from a leaf cutting, however, will produce a Mini-Me of the parent plant. Here's how you do that:

1. Cut a four- to six-inch portion of stem right above a leaf node (where two leaves emerge from the stem). Use a very sharp knife or pruners, and be sure to cut at an angle.

2. Cut off any extra leaves, leaving only the top few, and place the stem in a jar or vase of water. Make sure none of the leaves are in the water, as they will rot.

3. Keep your rooting plant somewhere warm but out of direct light, and add more water as it is absorbed or evaporates.

4. When the roots are an inch or two long, move your cutting to a pot filled with moist soil. The roots should be planted an inch below the soil surface and gently patted into place. Keep the soil consistently moist as your brand-new plant takes root in the pot.

Whichever way you get that baby coleus, as it grows up, give it proper coleus care: bright light (though it can survive in partial shade, too), damp soil at all times, and a nice spring fertilizer.

Rex begonia, another favorite foliage plant rated as "easy" to get in the propagation mood, is a hybrid plant like the coleus; you'll have to grow it from a leaf cutting to get a matching kind of leaf pattern. Though there are several types of begonias (rex is not the flowering kind you see in summer-front-porch container gardens), this one really is the king, with dazzling red, maroon, purple, silver, and green leaf patterns. You can select a leafy stem from a fabulously patterned parent plant and root it in water, just like with the coleus. If you want several new begonias at once, however, opt for a leaf cutting rooted directly from the plant's leaves:

1. Cut a single leaf from the base of the plant and remove its stalk.
2. Slash the underside of the leaf all the way through, right along its primary vein.
3. Pin the leaf directly to a pot filled with compost, slashed side down. Keep it warm and moist, and baby plants will start to grow straight from each slash in the leaf. A whole rex begonia garden from one leaf!
4. Gently separate the baby plants and give each its own new pot and soil to grow in. Or you can keep them together to get a fuller, bushier forest of begonias.

Now that your begonia family is growing, give them medium light (they can survive in lower light, but young ones will want more brightness) and an airy, lightweight soil in a shallow pot. Water when the top inch of soil is dry and try to keep that moisture off the leaves, which are known for

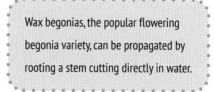

Wax begonias, the popular flowering begonia variety, can be propagated by rooting a stem cutting directly in water.

getting infected by a powdery mildew when too wet. Use a weak, diluted fertilizer to keep their soil replenished. Your young rex begonias will never be huge—it is not in their nature, no matter how they are grown—but they will brighten up terrariums and small indoor containers.

Some master propagators call for using rooting hormone to make the whole procedure go faster, whether with coleus, begonia, or any other houseplant. This technique is only necessary if you plan to be a frequent breeder or can offer less than ideal conditions. For a small indoor garden, stick with the basics first.

Branching Out

Propagating plants is certainly a less expensive tactic to expand your indoor garden, but it can also be a lovely and meaningful way to share a little green love with friends and family.

"If people get cuttings from their mom's plants or a neighbor's, they will always remember who they got that cutting from," says Matt Kostelnick of Ambius. "People are really impacted by plants."

Crystal Desi of Cactus Moon is among the many plant nursery owners who propagate their own crops to sell to customers. Selling the succulents and cacti that Desi grows from leaf cuttings is an ideal way to grow her business, but also a way to share a little piece of herself. Some of her progeny are passed down from plants she inherited from her grandmother, a farmer and collector of rare succulents.

A plant with a story brings that extra personal touch to your home. Some plants—for example, the popular string of pearls Desi propagates at home—carry a small chapter in a longer narrative of generations of plant lovers.

String of pearls is that delightful succulent that looks more like an overflowing cup of green peas than any necklace of oyster irritation. It's green, for one thing, and that isn't something one usually anticipates in a pearl. But in this pearl, it's perfect. How many plants have perfectly spherical leaves? Its stems grow in long, trailing strings just made for a trim:

- Select a string of pearls to cut, usually one you were planning to prune anyway. You will need to remove some of the leaves (the pearls) near the cut end to make sure you have at least one inch of stem to plant.
- Set the cutting aside for twenty-four hours for calluses to form over the cuts.
- Use a moistened succulent or cactus potting mix. Prepare a small hole in the potting mixture and tuck the cut end of the stem inside. Pat the mix gently into place around it.
- No watering! Place the string of pearls somewhere warm and not too bright, and leave it alone for two to three weeks. If any leaves start to pucker, then you can add water.
- Give it a light tug. Does it resist? That means it's rooting. Your plant is ready for water at this stage, but make sure you let it get dry to at least an inch below the surface before you water again; those are the succulent rules.

- Succulents from cuttings grow slowly at first, but it won't be too many more weeks before tiny new teardrop-shaped leaves begin to appear and then grow into fully formed round pearls.
- Return the favor: when your newly formed string of pearls is mature enough to produce its own long strands, share a cutting with someone special to you to pass along a little piece of precious green.

Now, those are some pearls you'll be proud to clutch. String together your own story from the plants that you acquire as cuttings: Your mother's spider plant. Your grandmother's philodendron. Your old roommate's aloe. Your second cousin's boyfriend's aunt's hairdresser's snake plant. These are rare pearls to collect indeed.

To Love, Honor, and Houseplant

Ryan and Meriel Lesseig started their Air Plant Design Studio after discovering how beautifully air plants amplified their own wedding flower displays, in bouquets, table settings, corsages, et cetera. They now offer their air plant stock for others' weddings or events as a living memory of a special day—how many wedding flowers will continue to bloom as anniversaries roll by?

The Lesseigs rely on propagation to grow their collection, but the process is a little different. Leaf cuttings grow roots; air plants grow pups.

Before you start picturing a cocker spaniel springing from your tillandsia, these pups, like those that form on the more familiar types of bromeliads we covered in chapter 6, are offsets of the mama plant that appear under its leaves when it is finished blooming. When the little pup is about half its parent's size, you can gently pull it away (if it resists, it's not ready to leave its mama yet) and raise it as a delightful symbol of your green thumb or pass it along to friends and family.

PROPAGATION OUTREACH

Now that you know how easy it is to propagate plants, you may start to peruse friends' and neighbors' indoor gardens with that same gleam in your eye with which Dr. Frankenstein regarded a cemetery: "If only I could get a cutting of that."

Please ask permission before snipping a stem from someone's plant. You don't want people hiding their houseplants when you come over the way they hide the good silver from that one kleptomaniac aunt.

Conversely, if someone asks you for a cutting, why not just say yes? Give a gift to the earth and grow more plants.

Here's a beautiful story of plant propagation used for the greater good: the showy lady's slipper. This is a type of dainty white-and-rose-colored orchid native to the woods of New England that was facing extinction in the wild. The late Dr. Bill Ballard, a renowned biology professor and researcher, started pollinating wild specimens and then harvesting their seeds to propagate them in his home. His background in embryology made him the ideal guardian for a species that must be grown not just from seed, but from a seed that germinates only in a certain kind of fungus, which is hard to replicate at home. A visit to his house found lady's slippers in various stages of growth along windowsills and especially in the bathroom, where the delicate bog natives had a special home in the bathtub. When his collection had grown, Dr. Ballard returned them to the wild, planting them in preserved bogs and wetlands where they would be protected and continue to grow and propagate on their own.

This is the ultimate in houseplant propagation, rescuing a plant species diminished and suffering from human environmental takeover, and making an indoor gardening effort an act of conservation, a small pink-and-white gesture of beauty.

Your home is your sanctuary. And whether you're happy with some fresh herbs and a nice desk succulent, or want to redesign your bedroom around a hanging garden headboard and share your shower with a Boston fern, plants are a way to transform your house into a home. They're an air-filtering gift, a stress reducer, an idea stimulator, a special memory, and an expression of your personal style.

Most of all: Houseplants make you happy.

And, armed with your new tips for indoor gardening success—from correctly draining pots and identifying light availability, to humidity regulation and watering techniques—you're prepared to make them happy, too.

Just don't put the cactus in the bathroom.

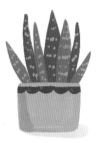

Acknowledgments

A special thank-you to all the indoor gardening experts who helped this book grow:

Julie Bawden-Davis, founder and publisher of HealthyHouseplants.com, a resource website for creating indoor gardens.

Crystal Desi, owner of Cactus Moon Market (cactusmoonmarket.com), a succulent specialty store in Tampa, Florida.

Matt Kostelnick, senior horticulturalist with Ambius (ambius.com), an indoor landscaping company serving commercial spaces.

Ryan and Meriel Lesseig, owners of Air Plant Design Studio (air-plants.com), a national premium air plant supplier.

Joyce Mast, in-house gardening expert "Plant Mom" at Bloomscape.com, a national online houseplant greenhouse.

Mary Beth Shaddix, a plant writer (marybethshaddix.com) and owner of Maple Valley Nursery (maplevalleynurseryllc.com) in Birmingham, Alabama.

Index

Index

M

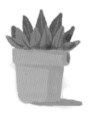

About the Author

Emily L. Hay Hinsdale is a freelance writer, an enthusiastic cook, a dedicated traveler, a determined pedestrian, and a lifelong gardener.

About the Illustrator

Loni Harris specializes in hand-lettering and florals and has had artwork with major US retailers such as Walmart, Target, Home Depot, and Staples. She loves hiking, working on her farm, and binge-watching while sketching.